D0775589

REAL
BODYBUILDING

Muscle Truth from 25 Years in the Trenches

RON HARRIS

authorHOUSE®

AuthorHouse™
1663 Liberty Drive, Suite 200
Bloomington, IN 47403
www.authorhouse.com
Phone: 1-800-839-8640

© 2008 Cover image by Per Bernal.

First published by AuthorHouse 8/4/2008

ISBN: 978-1-4389-0085-8 (sc)

Printed in the United States of America
Bloomington, Indiana

This book is printed on acid-free paper.

CONTENTS

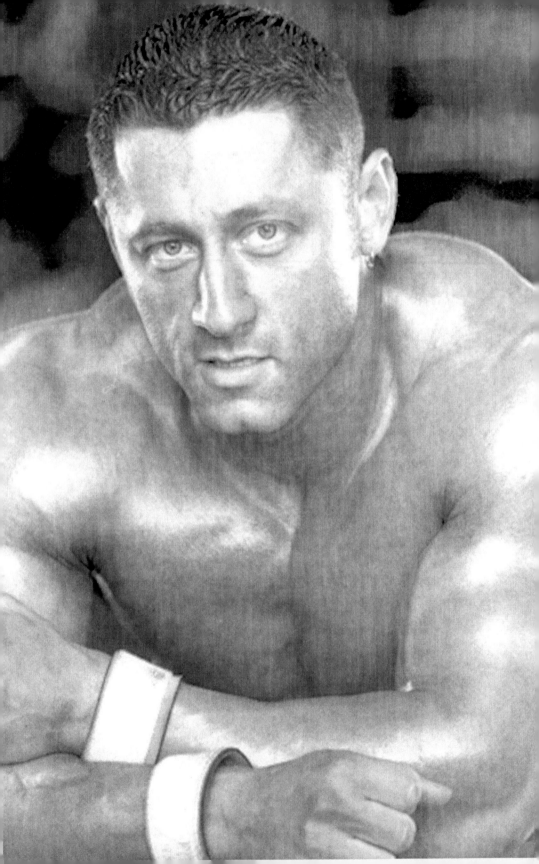

INTRODUCTION

Though this is not a book about me, I do feel it appropriate to share some of my background if I am asking you to accept me as someone who knows what he is talking about in the world of bodybuilding. I was born in September of 1969 and raised in the Boston suburb of Waltham, Massachusetts. From a very early age it was clear that I was not developing at the same rate as my peers, physically. My classmates, even the girls, all towered over me. It didn't matter that intellectually; I was fairly advanced, especially with regards to vocabulary and reading comprehension (I taught myself how to read at the age of three, somehow). If anything, that made me an even more attractive target for bullies, since I made them more aware of their own limited brainpower. In class, I was the teacher's pet and a straight-A student, outside I was picked on and occasionally beaten. The worst time was in eighth grade when two big thugs who each outweighed me by a solid thirty pounds did the cat-and-mouse toying thing, taking turns pummeling me for a half-hour before stuffing my bloodied, scrawny little body in a locker and slamming it shut. One of them became a State Police officer and blew his brains out with a .38 at the age of twenty-two. The other one has been in and out of jail several times and is an alcoholic. That's poetic justice for you right there.

So even by the time I was nine or ten years old, I had the fantasy of getting big and strong and being so tough that any bully, no matter how much of a bad-ass, would cower in fear of my kicking his punk ass. That was the main thing in my pre-adolescent mind, to no longer be someone who was picked on. My early role models were wrestlers in the old 70's WWF before it went mainstream; guys like Hulk Hogan, "Superstar" Billy Graham, Tony Atlas, Jimmy "Superfly" Snuka, Ken Patera, and Ivan Putski. A bit later in the early and mid 80's there was a Texas wrestler named Kerry Von Erich, who probably had the best physique ever seen in pro wrestling. This guy was young, he had rock-star good looks and hair, and he was built like a heavyweight bodybuilder. This girl Nancy LeBlanc I had a crush on for a few years was enthralled with Kerry. I sure wanted to be Kerry (sadly, he was another suicide). Even though it was all an act and these guys were just playing the roles of supremely tough, fearless macho sons of bitches, the powerful and heavily muscled bodies were quite real. I didn't have any idea at the time that weight training was their secret to looking like that.

Lifting weights was something two of my older brothers had done for a short time in junior high. We had different dads so the genetics weren't exactly the same, but I remember Roger, eight years older than I, building little peaked biceps and a bit of a beefy chest. My dad, a mail carrier named Alan Davenport Harris who passed away when I was sixteen, also did dumbbell concentration curls in the basement on a rotting old stuffed chair that stank of mildew, and the stuffing of which had mostly fallen out over the years. He always used the same rusted-together dumbbell, which weighed 43 ½ pounds (I weighed it), and only did that one exercise. And looking back now, I think his form was pretty bad. But whenever I heard that clinging of the dumbbell moving around in the dank cellar air downstairs, I raced down and sat quietly in the corner watching (he didn't like any interruptions). I used to think, *yeah, my dad is pretty tough and strong. He lifts weights. I'm gonna lift weights when I'm old enough.* Probably the final catalyst was being inspired by the transformation of Nancy Leblanc's older brother, Jerry. Jerry had a bodybuilder phase in between his Marine Corps Junior ROTC phase and his punk rocker period. I don't think he even trained a full two years before giving up, but managed to build a little physique by age sixteen that was like a miniature Frank Zane. And damn, was he cut. The kid always had a six-pack and all these thick, gnarly veins running up and down his arms. Jerry was the first genetic freak I ever met. I was so jealous, especially when girls would swoon over him and ask to feel his arms, squealing with giggles when they touched his bulging biceps. His little pile of *Muscle and Fitness* magazines were the first I ever saw, and I recall being completely overwhelmed at the bodies of the guys like Samir Bannout, Bertil Fox, and Tom Platz, thinking they just couldn't possibly be real. And suddenly a new factor had entered the picture. At almost fourteen (I looked about twelve), I had barely started puberty but already the hormones had me thinking about girls and sex 24-7. But being 4-11 and 90 pounds, as well as shy, meant I was perfectly invisible to females. Huh, if I got me some muscles, the chicks would be lining up to get to me, I figured in my quite immature estimation. One day I woke up and simply knew the right moment had arrived. It was time to start getting serious about lifting weights.

I had a Marcy bench and weights that I had asked for and got for Christmas in seventh grade. I had expected to double in size from the moment I started using it, and got discouraged right away when that failed to transpire. The workouts were few and far between after the first few days I had it. Now I returned to it with a new purpose, closely following the illustrated chart that had come with it and getting a very rudimentary idea of which exercises worked which muscles. I worked on mainly my chest and arms, though I would also throw in some leg extensions and one-arm rows. After a year of this, the results were far from stunning. I think I grew two inches in height and was up to a whopping 100 pounds. At the start of tenth grade my friend Paul Poirier and I decided to train together in his attic three times a week after school. He was my first training partner, and man, did we have some good workouts for two guys who had only the vaguest idea what we were doing. We always started with the bench press, and Paul at the time was far larger and stronger than me. After that would come curls, maybe some overhead presses, plus weird things we would invent like holding a ten-pound plate in each hand with arms out straight as long as we could. Paul would pull a ski cap over his eyes as he believed this increased his pain threshold. The dimly-lit attic was a sauna of dry heat in the summer, and cold enough to see your breath plume out in the late fall, winter, and into the early spring. Paul had a record player in there and only a few records that were deemed worthy of lifting to. They were AC/DC's *Back in Black*, Aerosmith's *Toys in the Attic*, and of course, as every white boy owned in those days, *Led Zeppelin* IV.

There were also a few classic movies that deserve to be mentioned, as they also motivated millions of other young men to train – many of you reading this, I bet. First were the *Rocky* movies, more specifically the big training montage near the end of each right before the big fight. You couldn't help but feel the adrenaline rush as that theme music started blasting – *Gonna Fly Now*, *Eye of the Tiger*, whatever – and Rocky would be running, lifting weights, doing sit-ups while getting punched in the gut between reps, one-arm push-ups. His face was a grimace of pain, sweat ran down in rivers, and you knew this guy was working as hard as a human being possibly could. Didn't we all have little bursts of similar training after we saw these movies? Stallone went on to do the *Rambo* movies, running around with his shirt off and shooting big M-60 machine guns. But the real man when it comes to motivation was Arnold Schwarzenegger. I was babysitting for my older sister Jackie one night around 1979 at her apartment when *Pumping Iron* came on PBS. Though I was only nine or ten, seeing Arnold and the other top bodybuilders of the 70's training, joking around, and competing was a total shock to my system. It was the first time I ever made the connection between weights and muscles. Every time I saw Arnold after that, in movies like *Conan the Barbarian*, *The Terminator*, and *Commando*, I always remembered the 'secret' to that incredibly muscular body on screen.

I kept training, but the whole bodybuilding thing didn't really begin until my first semester at UC Santa Barbara in fall of 1987. I picked up my first issue of *Flex* and all at once I was mesmerized. I turned into a bodybuilding fanatic in a matter of days after that. True, for well over a year I was convinced from reading a couple books by Arthur Jones and Ellington Darden that Nautilus machines were the only legitimate tools to train with, but I still made progress. I started competing in 1989 in the ANBC, a lifetime drug-free organization based in Rhode Island, and had transferred back east to Emerson College in Boston, a communications school. Toward the end of 1989, while working as an 'instructor' at a health club in Newton, MA, I met my wife Janet and we have been inseparable ever since. Emerson had an LA Program for seniors where we would take a couple classes while interning for a company in the entertainment industry. I knew I wanted to go back to California after having been away for over two years, but I wasn't sure where I wanted to intern. Having the internship set up was a prerequisite for the program. I was thinking maybe the *American Gladiators* show would be cool to work for.

I was in a gym that no longer exists, the supremely hardcore Powerhouse Gym in Watertown, MA, with one of the Emerson film department's 16mm cameras, working on my student film. The title was "All Natural," and all it really consisted of was footage of a couple local natural bodybuilders working out and posing with rock music in the background. It was pretty lame now that I think about it. But Vinny Greco, the gym owner, suggested I send a copy to Lou Zwick, producer of the *American Muscle Magazine* show on ESPN. For those of you who never saw it, it was a magazine-format show that had bodybuilding contest coverage, workout segments, profiles, cooking, nutrition, and more. It ran from 1987 until 2002. Despite bodybuilding being such a marginal sport, it was the longest-running show on the network aside from *Sportscenter*. To list all the top bodybuilders who appeared on the show would take a whole chapter. Let's just say that pretty much everyone who was anyone in bodybuilding was on it at one time or another, many of them long before they were famous. Lou had a knack for spotting both competitive and marketing potential and discovered quite a few stars. I put a demo reel together and sent it off to LA. Lou liked the fact that I was both an avid bodybuilder myself and also had a sense of how to shoot and edit, the basic skills needed to work in television production. Soon after that, I packed everything I owned into my Mustang and headed west to LA where my transformation into a complete meathead shortly began in January of 1991.

Within a week I had joined Gold's Gym in Venice and was driving across LA to train there four times a week. In June, I went back home and got married and brought Janet back. By that time school was over, but I had been hired as the show's Associate Producer. I advanced in the company the old-fashioned way – by filling the positions of two older guys who had quit. At twenty-one years old, I was writing and directing most of the segments on the one-hour monthly show. Over the next seven years the show was my life, and I owe it and Lou credit for meeting all the athletes in bodybuilding and fitness, the officials, contest promoters, supplement company honchos, photographers, and magazine staff. I went to all the big amateur and pro shows and became part of the little family that makes up the bodybuilding industry. In the beginning I was quite intimidated by almost everybody and everything, but over time I became more comfortable with my job and gained confidence.

At the same time, I started writing for the magazines in my spare time. The first was *Ironman*, then I got hooked up with *Musclemag*. There were many other smaller publications I was only too eager to contribute to as well in the early years. I also never stopped training and competing, which vexed Lou to no end. Being a bodybuilder is not very compatible with working in television production. Most of the people in that world often work very long hours and only break for meals perhaps once every six hours or so. It was a struggle to keep my schedule of eating every two hours, but I was determined. I arrived in LA at 185 pounds and grew to 230 (natural and with a good amount of fat) within two years. Eventually, I got sick of the job, and when Lou found out I was secretly interviewing for similar positions at shows like *Entertainment Tonight* and *Inside Edition*, he fired me. Immediately I felt freed from a heavy burden. From that day on I would be my own boss, and by God, nobody was going to tell me when I could eat or go to the gym again!

After working for about eighteen months as a personal trainer, my writing assignments became steady and plentiful enough for me to at last become a full-time magazine writer. Janet and I had a daughter Marisa, born in 1994, and then our son Christian came along in 1999. With no real reason to remain in LA any more, we moved back to Boston in the fall of 2000. After all, as long as I have a computer, a telephone, and Internet access, I can do my job from anywhere. Now I am one of the top writers in bodybuilding, with over two thousand articles published in around two-dozen different magazines and web sites since 1992. I started writing for Steve Blechman's *Muscular Development* in early 2002, and got in at a very good time, as this magazine has been rocketing upward in circulation and page count ever since. And thanks to Steve, I am back in the press pit at some of the big shows again for the first time since I stopped working for the ESPN show.

Of course, I still train and still compete, more than twenty years after I picked up my first weight. I don't exactly look like Ronnie Coleman and I don't have a collection of cool-sounding titles, but I love the sport and do it purely for fun and the challenge of constantly improving on my previous best. I am a bodybuilder and I will always be a bodybuilder because it's in my blood. It's not even about what you look like or how many pictures you have in the magazines or on the Internet, it's about what's in your heart. In my heart I am a bodybuilder. Lifting heavy weights, getting a pump, checking out your development and progress in the mirror – these are things the average person will never understand, but to we bodybuilders they are part of our lives. If you know that bodybuilding is a way of life and an attitude more so than it is a sport, then this book is definitely for you.

We are going to be covering a very wide range of topics, and I am warning you right now that you will be surprised, shocked, maybe even angered about some of the things you will read. This is especially true if you have read a few of the fluffy, generic books on bodybuilding targeted toward beginners. Those books give you a sanitized version of bodybuilding and what it takes to be a great bodybuilder, and often they sugarcoat the truth if not gloss right over it completely. That's not me. I am an honest person, which doesn't always make me very popular and sometimes gets me in trouble, but I can't help my nature. This book will have not a speck of bullshit. I am going to give it to you straight up, based on all my experiences as a bodybuilder and as part of the bodybuilding industry over the years. It's going to be real, it's going to be hardcore, and it's going to open up your eyes. Are you ready? Can you handle the truth? If so, let's rock and roll, people!

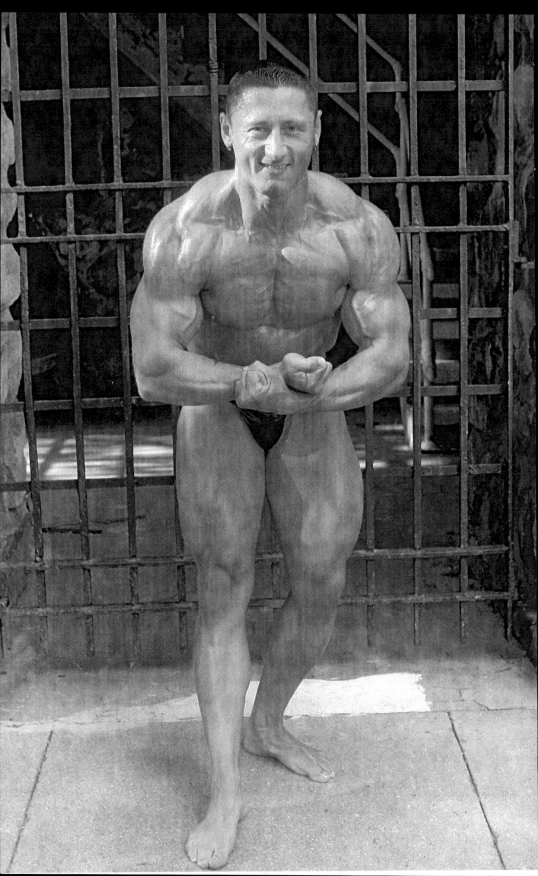

01

SO, YOU WANNA BE A HARDCORE BODYBUILDER?

What Is Hardcore, Exactly?

The term "hardcore" is used a lot in bodybuilding, but is rarely defined. Many people seem to equate being hardcore with using steroids, though one certainly doesn't have to juice it up to meet the criteria. I, for example, was thoroughly hardcore years before a needle ever sank into my ass and delivered my first dose of Sustanon back in late 1997. Hardcore is really a way to describe someone who is fully committed to bodybuilding. We are not just flirting with bodybuilding, we are married to it with divorce as unlikely a possibility as it was in the USA fifty years ago. A hardcore bodybuilder has decided to dedicate their lives to developing the best physique they are capable of. This is not a conditional goal with a time limit, as in "I will do everything right for two years, and if after that I don't look like a pro I will quit." No, because bodybuilding is a never-ending process – a journey and not a destination.

Bodybuilding is something that requires far more commitment than nearly any other sport or pastime I can think of. Anybody can meet up with their softball league a couple times a week and play with the boys while throwing back a few beers and call themselves an athlete, but to legitimately call yourself a bodybuilder means that everything you do from the moment you wake up to the time you go back to sleep needs to serve your bodybuilding goals. While this doesn't mean you have to give up working and having friends and family relationships, it does mean that nutrition, training, and supplementation are always on your mind. More on the specifics of that in a little while.

Do you have to compete to be hardcore? No, you don't have to at all. But to those of us who do compete, there is an extra measure of respect we reserve for others who do. Competing means that you have taken your level of commitment to a higher level than most ever will. Anybody can train to gain mass or lose fat just for his or her own satisfaction, but to compete means that you have chosen a specific day to put it all together to the best of your ability. On the day of this show, you will have worked diligently for months of training and dieting to arrive with the most muscular package you are capable of, and then you will stand next to others who have done the same wearing nothing but tiny posing briefs and a coat of oil. Under the bright stage lights in front of a crowd and a panel of judges, you will be evaluated and compared to the others until the judges have put the lineup in the order of placement they feel is correct, looking at factors such as size, shape, condition, symmetry, and presentation. Anyone who thinks this whole process is easy has never tried it. Many hardcore bodybuilders never compete or even diet down to a very low bodyfat, preferring to simply lift heavy and eat as they wish without ever having to suffer through the physical and mental agonies of dieting down. That is their choice. Yet others will diet down, usually in the summer, as an annual practice to show off what they worked hard to build in the cold weather months, but have no desire to enter a contest. Looking like a ripped, muscular stallion and getting attention and compliments are better to them than any trophy or title.

Finally, some seem to think that there is a direct correlation between your size and how hardcore you truly are. It's a form of elitism, wherein those who are 250, 300 pounds or even heavier feel superior to their smaller and lighter peers. One man who is himself well over six foot and nearly 400 pounds (and who has never been seen without a baggy T-shirt or sweatshirt, I might add) told me in an e-mail that "anyone who weighs less than 300 pounds can't be training very hard."

They can go on believing this bunk if they choose to, but it is out of step with reality. We all have very different genetics, which is the subject of the following chapter. Let's just say that a heavy-boned man who starts training at 6-2 and already weighing a husky 240 pounds is going to weigh a lot more eventually than a light-framed guy who begins working out at 5-4 and 110 pounds. I don't define hardcore by appearance, although maxing out on your individual potential is a vital component. If you have worked hard and come a long way from where you started in terms of size and strength, you are hardcore regardless of whether you weigh 180 or 340 pounds.

But most hardcore bodybuilders do want to get bigger, no matter how much or little space they currently occupy on planet Earth. Someone who is hardcore doesn't start training with the vague idea of 'putting on a little bit of size' or 'toning up.' No, we are the ones who will always struggle and scrape to get just a little more muscle, even if everyone around us assures us that we are quite big enough already. Even if we constantly hear we are too big, in our minds we still aren't. How big is too big? To the truly hardcore man or woman, there is no such thing. Ronnie Coleman, Markus Ruhl, Jay Cutler, these guys are all role models for their outrageously developed physiques.

Are Hardcore Bodybuilders A Little Crazy?

One thing I think nearly all hardcore bodybuilders have in common is that we are a little nuts. I always noticed there are two distinct kinds of bodybuilders, generally speaking. The first is the former star athlete, someone who excelled at sports like football, wrestling, or gymnastics, and makes the transition to bodybuilding as a logical progression when their days at the other sports come to an end. These also tend to be the more genetically gifted among bodybuilders, as many of the same physical traits that lend themselves to success in these other sports translate well to developing an extremely muscular physique. This group is in the minority among bodybuilders, perhaps making up about five percent of us. Then there are the rest of us.

Most bodybuilders take to the activity based almost entirely on insecurity. In my case, I was insecure because of my small size and hoped to find respect and admiration in a larger body. The 'short man' or Napoleon complex is quite common, particularly in bodybuilders of less than average height (luckily for me, at least I did grow to 5-9 eventually). Others began because they felt like social outcasts, and believed that becoming muscular would help them assimilate and fit in. I am sure a lot of bodybuilders were also physically and verbally abused as children, made by bad parents to feel worthless and pathetic. For them, becoming a bodybuilder is a means to validate their very existence and prove that they are somebody. I think the victim mentality in general drives many a tortured young man or woman to pick up weights and attempt to forge a muscular suit of armor to protect and insulate them from any who would seek to harm them. I certainly don't have a psychology degree, but it's not hard to figure out the various motives that would spur a man or woman to devote their lives to a regimented system of eating and training. And we can't leave out sex, or more specifically, the desire to be more sexually attractive. In my hormone-soaked adolescent mind, my terror of girls and inability to communicate with them with any degree of confidence would instantly be washed away when I built a muscular physique. To some extent that proved true, though my assumption that muscles were irresistible to all females was later found to be wrong. We deal with this issue in more detail in a later chapter, as it does merit further discussion.

The Hardcore Life Of A Real Bodybuilder – Good And Bad

Before embarking on your quest to become a bodybuilder, it's important to know the positives and negatives of the lift you will be leading. First, the good stuff to look forward to. Obviously, your body will be much better than the average slob who doesn't take part in any physical activity. You will be stronger and have more lean muscle mass, and less fat than Joe or Jane Public. With this comes a sense of pride and enhanced self-esteem. You are a walking symbol of achievement through hard work, diligence, perseverance, and sacrifice. Everywhere you go, people will recognize you as being different from the crowd. Many members of the opposite sex (or same sex, depending on your preference, you may assume from here on in that this is inferred) will find you more attractive due to your sculpted body. If you are a man, you will be far less likely to be the target of bullying, a practice that some bullies continue their whole lives. Not that everyone will cower in fear from you, but any man is less likely to start a fight with a dude who is a lean 250 at six foot than he would if the potential victim was a skinny 5-6 and 120 pounds. If you eat clean food, do cardio as well as lift weights, and abstain from recreational drug or alcohol abuse, you will be far healthier than the average person.

Now, here are the bad parts about being a bodybuilder you should know. I would say the worst thing is that when a lot of people see you, they will automatically assume that your are dumb, vain, hostile, or all of the above. Much of this stems from simple jealousy. Most people have no control over their bodies – just look at how many grossly obese folks you see – and resent anyone who has mastered theirs through a significant application of willpower and dedication. In essence, we bodybuilders through nothing more than our appearance make these people more aware of their own terrible bodies and their failure to do anything to improve them. Think about how many overweight people are always trying new diets and yo-yoing up and down in weight. All they really need to do is combine a better eating approach with regular exercise, but they are too weak mentally to do so. Some members of the opposite sex will feel intimidated by you because you spend so much time exercising and pay such close attention to your diet, or perhaps even think you are dangerously obsessed with these. And know this – you do have to be obsessed with working out and eating right to be a real bodybuilder. You have to be consistent with your workouts and meals, meaning that no matter where you go or what the circumstance, you must always be sure you have access to the proper foods. It takes a lot of the spontaneity out of life, but that's a price we pay.

As for big muscles making you immune to hostile jerkoffs who love to start fights, that is not always the case. There will always be some asshole who will want to kick your ass to show his girlfriend that he's tougher than you, and he will usually be too drunk to care that you may outweigh him by fifty pounds and be able to toss him across the room like a football. I suppose the hardest reality of being a bodybuilder is that few who do not live the same lifestyle as you will ever understand or appreciate what it is you do. I recently read a quote that sums it up: "obsessed is a word the lazy use to describe the dedicated." Bodybuilders often have trouble maintaining romantic relationships with mates who do not live the muscle life. Very few people will think it is normal and productive to put as much importance on our bodies as we do, and breakups and divorce rates are rampant when muscleheads try to live with 'normal' people. The most doomed relationships seem to be the ones where the man is a bodybuilders and doesn't make much money. Often I hear of ultimatums where the man is forced to choose between giving up bodybuilding and finding a way to earn more cash, or else the woman is leaving. This is why we tend to gravitate toward others like us who understand our unique passion.

Where Will You Find Others Like You?

I know of only one place in this world where there actually is a fairly sizeable concentration of bodybuilders. This is the neighborhood of Los Angeles named Venice Beach, otherwise known as The Mecca to bodybuilders. While I doubt Moslems would appreciate the title, it is so dubbed because all hardcore bodybuilders simply must make the pilgrimage once in their lives. Venice Beach became known as Muscle Beach in the 1940's when pioneer bodybuilders like Armand Tanny, George Eiferman, and Steve Reeves went there to train in the outdoor weight pit. By the time the early Seventies rolled around, many of the top bodybuilders in the world lived there and trained in the original Gold's Gym. These were the "Pumping Iron" years, when at any given moment you might happen to see Arnold, Franco, Dave Draper, Frank Zane, Robby Robinson, Ken Waller, Bill Grant, or Mike Katz. Some of them, like Arnold and Franco, also liked to train at the newer outdoor weight pen, and they all liked to lay out on the grass and tan between their morning and late afternoon workouts.

Though most of those legends left the area, hundreds more champion and aspiring bodybuilders followed, certainly influenced by the idealized image they had of Venice after seeing *Pumping Iron*. In the late 70's, the first Gold's Gym shut down for good and a new, larger Gold's Gym opened up a couple blocks north on Hampton Drive. Within a couple years, this gym became the most famous in the world, and could claim among it s members the very elite of amateur and professional bodybuilding. To name them all here would take quite a while, but just a few of the more prominent members have been the Barbarian Brothers, Flex Wheeler, Chris Cormier, Aaron Baker, the late Lyle Alzado, Rick Valente, Lou Ferrigno, and Hulk Hogan. It became and remains a very popular location for magazine photo shoots and the nerve center of the bodybuilding world. Soon after, Joe Gold opened up the first World Gym less than a mile away, and this became the training headquarters for Arnold and many of the pre-1980's bodybuilding champions. Gold's Gym today has a circus-like atmosphere, the only place I know where nothing is shocking. You may see a 260-pound pro bodybuilder training next to a movie star, with a porn star or Kobe Bryant in opposite corners of one of the four huge rooms. You will see pro and amateur bodybuilders from all over the USA and the world who have come to Venice to make their fortune, or so they hope.

A couple blocks away is the restaurant you are most likely to run into any number of top bodybuilding stars, the Firehouse on Main Street. The menu caters to bodybuilders, with such meals as "The Bodybuilder Lunch" – half a roasted chicken, a large yam, and steamed vegetables. On the same block are two other restaurants with many bodybuilding patrons, Koo Koo Roo and Fresh to Go. You will also find retail stores with bodybuilding clothes and supplements, such as Hot Skins and Max Muscle, still on that same block. The outdoor weight pit was torn down and a much better equipped and aesthetically pleasing replacement was built in the early 1990's. You won't find many name bodybuilders there, as the lifters seem to be mostly heavily-tattooed, recently released LA County Jail inmates with an exhibitionistic streak looking to show off the muscles they built in the joint. Powerhouse Gym also opened up a new franchise next to Koo Koo Roo and across from the Firehouse, so you can see how this little area has become such a popular destination for bodybuilders. They come from all over the world to vacation in what can only be politely called a pretty run-down section of Los Angeles, just to soak in the atmosphere and gain inspiration for when they return home from this bodybuilder's paradise. Where else can you train where the stars of the sport train, eat where the stars eat, and rub elbows with men and women you have only seen before in magazines?

Quite a few bodybuilders move to Venice or a surrounding area like Santa Monica with the twin goals of becoming a pro bodybuilder and an actor, just like Arnold. Since the competition is fierce and any area only needs so many personal trainers, a majority of these men and women return to wherever they came from within a year or two. But do I recommend that you all visit Venice at least once every few years? Absolutely! If you are in an isolated part of the USA or somewhere else in the world where you are looked upon as a weirdo or a freak for your obsession with muscles, Venice will feel like the home you never had.

Another way to meet and mingle with our own kind is at the big bodybuilding contests and their accompanying expos. The huge one in the spring is the Arnold Schwarzenneger Classic, called 'the Arnold' for short, held every March in Columbus, Ohio. The Arnold has the most going on in terms of display booths, with nearly 500 at last count, and strongman contests, powerlifting, martial arts, dance, and cheerleading also taking place. In October, we have the Olympia Weekend, which has more or less found a permanent home in Las Vegas, a very appropriate locale for the circus atmosphere of bodybuilders, their fans, supporters, and groupies. There is also the USA Championships in Las Vegas every July, and the NPC Nationals in November in a different city each year. I can't leave out the New York Pro in New York City every May, or the mammoth FIBO convention in Germany in spring where all the European bodybuilding and fitness crowd converges. Ironically, you will run into a lot of the same people at all these events, not unlike how the Grateful Dead had a loyal group of Deadheads that followed their tours. The expos feature booths with companies in the realms of fitness clothing, supplements, exercise equipment, and lot of other assorted products and services catering to bodybuilders. Most of the booths have the athletes who endorse their products working there, meeting fans and selling photos. It's an easy way for fans to get a lot closer to their idols and actually meet them, rather than just watching them on stage. And for the guys, it's especially cool because many booths hire knockout young women wearing practically nothing to entice you over. The job of these women is to smile and be nice, no matter how big of a dork you are. I always say the real entertainment is the men and women walking around. You will never believe there are so many people with incredible physiques who you have never heard of and may never hear of. This is their chance to strut their stuff, so it isn't uncommon at the Arnold to see guys walking around in string tank tops and girls wearing not much more than a swimsuit covers – even though it's freezing cold outside with snow on the ground.

Basically, it's not hard to find other hardcore bodybuilders if you know when and where they get together, which isn't hard. We are much like a close-knit family, and it's amazing how few of us there really are once you have been around a while and have been to these big shows a few times. That's what's really special about being a hardcore bodybuilder. It takes a special breed of person to become one and remain one, and hence we stick together. I will leave you with a quote:

"Obsessed is a word the lazy use to describe the dedicated"
– Author Unknown.

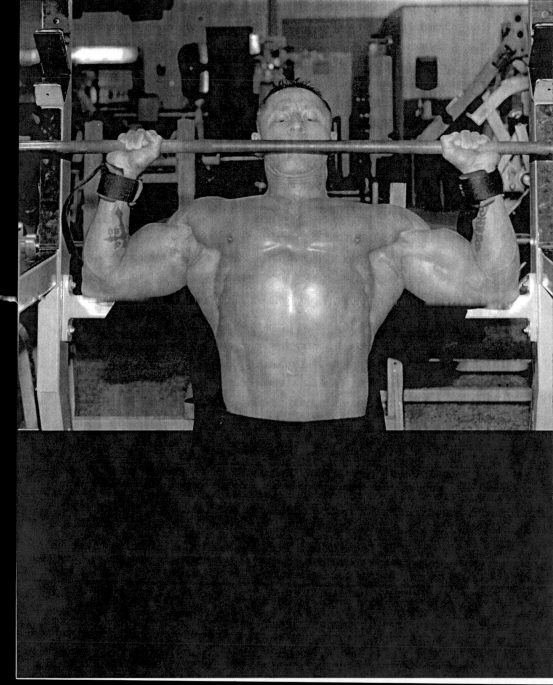

drove me to put on nearly a hundred pounds of muscle over the years, even though I still couldn't give any of the real stars of the sport a run for their money on stage. You can only hope to do that if you share the same physical gifts as they do which will allow you body to take on that incredible appearance eventually. Right, but just what types of gifts are we talking about?

What Are The Ideal Genetics For Bodybuilding?

Somatypes

Most people have an oversimplified version of what constitutes 'ideal' genetics for the sport of bodybuilding based on the three classic somatypes, or body types. These are mainly descriptions of bone structure, and the three broad categories are endomorph, ectomorph, and mesomorph. Endomorphs tend to have heavy bones, and hips that are wider than their shoulders - the typical pear shape. They gain fat easily. Some of them also gain muscle mass and strength easily. The vast majority of powerlifting champions and World's Strongest Man competitors have endomorphic tendencies. Endos don't tend to make great bodybuilders because the heavy bone structure does not lend itself to an aesthetically pleasing physique. Think about it, you could take most of the 320-pound linemen in the NFL and diet them down to three percent bodyfat. Though they would technically carry more mass than most bodybuilders, it would look big and clunky, like a shapeless blob.

Next up are the ectomorphs, lighter boned folks who often have both narrow shoulders and narrow hips. Though not always tall, many taller men and women fall into this category. Longer than average limbs are another giveaway. Nearly every player in the NBA could be classified as an ectomorph. Gaining weight of any kind is difficult for them, yet they are blessed with a naturally fast metabolism that often lets them stay very lean yet eat all kinds of junk food regularly. There have been very few ectomorphs who became bodybuilding champions. A rare example is Flex Wheeler, though he still couldn't be called a pure ectomorph. The challenge for ectos is filling out those long limbs. When a man is six-foot four and his arms are as long as a shorter bodybuilder's legs, he basically has to get those arms as big around as the other guy's legs for them to look impressive. There have only been a handful of men over six foot two who ever built enough muscle mass to compete as pro bodybuilders: Lou Ferrigno, Rolf Moeller, Quincy Taylor are three. Again, none of them would be considered ectomorphs, because they did possess structural attributes of the mesomorph.

And now let's talk about that lucky mesomorph. The bone structure is commonly called 'athletic' by mainstream people, characterized by wide shoulders and a narrow hips. The arms and legs are proportioned just right, neither too short or too long. When the ancient Greeks and Romans were sculpting their visions of the ideal body, they were chipping away marble blocks to reveal pure mesomorphs. Mesomorphs tend to gain muscle easily without getting fat, and the mass looks ten times as impressive as it would on an endomorph's frame because the joints are smaller. Open up a bodybuilding magazine on the newsstand, and every single man and woman you see is a mesomorph. Arnold, Lee Haney, Dorian, Ronnie – all mesos to the core.

Joint Size

This gives you the bare minimum idea of the genetic traits needed to be a champion bodybuilder, but it's only a start. I mentioned joint size, and it bears further discussion. In bodybuilding, the smaller your joints are, such as the knees, wrists, and elbows, the better. Tiny joints create the illusion of bigger muscles. Think about someone like Flex Wheeler hitting a front double biceps pose. Flex has such small wrists and elbows that the arm muscles seem to come out of nowhere. They look perfectly round. His thighs sweep out from tiny knees and lead up to tiny hips. A man with much thicker joints can have just as much muscle or more than Flex, but you wouldn't look twice at him if he hit the same pose. That's why I never pay much heed when Internet tough guys brag about weighing 280 and having 22-inch arms. Numbers mean jack shit in a visual sport like bodybuilding. Most of these clowns look like wrestlers or football linemen. No, I take that back, because professional wrestling now has a lot of very good physiques. I remember hanging around at the 1991 Mr. Olympia contest at the Disney World Dolphin Hotel, watching one of the *Friday the 13th* sequels in a lobby with Nimrod King, who was a pro for about ten minutes. He was telling me that when he dieted down to contest condition, his wrists got smaller. I remember thinking, what a Nimrod! Even then I knew that bones don't change once you are an adult. Nimrod had some of the tiniest wrists and joints in general I ever saw on a man carrying so much muscle.

Muscle insertions

After joint size, muscle insertions and shape have to be looked at. Muscle insertions determine to what degree a specific muscle can be developed. The easiest examples to illustrate this are the biceps and the calves. Your own biceps are either short, average, or long in length. You can figure this out in two seconds by flexing your bicep with the forearm and upper arm at a right angle. How much space is there in between the end of your biceps and your elbow? If there's a lot of room there, your bi's are short, like Albert Beckles or Chris Dickerson's. If there's about an inch of space, consider your muscle length average. If there's no room at all and your biceps muscle is jammed right up against the elbow joint like the great Sergio Oliva's was, congratulations! You have long biceps. Having long muscles means that you have more muscle cells to work with and increase the size of. The calves are the same way, with the two extremes being high and low calves. Flex your calf and see where the muscle ends on its way to your ankle. If it stops not too far down from your knee, sorry dude, you are stuck with high calves. You can beat the crap out of them but they will always be a weak point on your body. If they go way down like the cows of Tom Platz, Mike Matarazzo, Roger Stewart, Dorian Yates, or Paul DeMayo, you are in luck. In fact, you probably have nice calves without even training them. Ironically, some of the lowest calf insertions I have ever seen have been on grossly overweight men and women, and the mere act of supporting all that bodyweight while they waddle around has given some of them calves most bodybuilders would die for. Every muscle on your body inserts wherever it has been programmed to end up by your particular DNA. All this nonsense about preacher curls being able to 'fill in' short biceps is nothing but wishful thinking. To look like one of today's top bodybuilders, you must have small joints and long muscles. But wait, there's more!

Muscle Shape

The final physical ingredient required to build an elite physique such as those displayed by men like Ronnie Coleman, Jay Cutler, and Victor Martinez, is optimal muscle shape. To be exact, round muscle shape is what you want to have. The muscles should sweep off the bone and flare out and away. This is the only genetic prerequisite that can't be assessed until you have built some muscle, because it would be latent until the muscle grew a substantial amount from is untrained state. The easiest way to think about muscle shape is again with the biceps. You either have a peaked shape to them or you don't, depending on what your genetic code was set for. No amount of preacher curls or concentration curls will bring out a peak on your biceps unless you were going to have one anyway. A good example is Sergio Oliva. Sergio had some of the biggest arms ever seen in bodybuilding, but they looked like footballs. His biceps had no peak to them at all. Meanwhile, his rival Arnold had some of the best peaks to his biceps even to this day. Did Arnold do some secret exercises to bring those peaks out that Sergio missed? No, all you need to do is take a look at pictures of Arnold when he was just starting to train at around age fourteen. Small as his arms were compared to what they would become, the peaks on his biceps were already starting to show. Muscle shape, just like muscle length, is a factor that cannot be changed.

Great Genetics Can't Be Hidden For Long

Exceptional genetics become obvious quickly once most bodybuilders start training. I bet if you think back, you all know at least one or two guys back when you were a teenager who would have made great bodybuilders. As soon as these types start to weight train, their bodies practically explode with muscle. There was a black kid at my school named Paul who was in the grade ahead of me. I remember one time when a friend and I were messing around in the weight room of the Waltham Boy's Club when we were in eighth grade, Paul was this tall, very skinny kid with a sunken chest. His clavicles were wide thinking back, but at that time all we noticed was how thin he was. Me and my buddy Bart chuckled at Bart's whispered nickname for him, 'stringbean.' About a year later, I went back to the Boy's Club and again started trying to put some size on, and there was Stringbean. In the year I had been gone, Paul had been spending a couple hours after school every day, doing nothing but flat bench presses and curls. I almost didn't believe this was the same kid, because now he had thick, round arms with veins wrapping all around them, a beefy chest, and solid shoulders. Some of you are thinking, steroids! No fucking way. Paul came from a family of very modest means (I am almost sure they were on welfare), and he would never have been able to afford even the smallest cycle. I talked to him a few times and he ate just like all of us, junk food here and there with maybe one good meal every day at dinner. And let's not forget, he was training the same muscle groups every day for five or six days in a row (he took Sundays off, I know at one point he was very religious). The other kid I knew like this was Jorge Orta, the first Cuban I ever met, many years before I married one. I went to school with Jorge from seventh grade all the way to high school graduation, and even at age thirteen his nickname was Conan. He had the type of muscle thickness at that age that many guys never get in their lives. By ninth or tenth grade he could bench press 405 at a weight of only about 180 (he was pretty short, maybe 5' 6").

I have had the opportunity to interview literally thousands of top amateur and professional bodybuilders over the years, and a common thread ties them all together. Though not all were muscular before they started lifting weights (some were – Vince Taylor and Don Youngblood both had 18-inch arms before they ever touched a weight), as soon as they started working out the muscle just sprouted like weeds. I talk to a lot of them who have won their first contest within six months or a year of training. Some guys tell me they gained fifty or sixty pounds of muscle in their first year. Others had nice shape from the beginning and had to work harder and longer for the size to come, but within a year or two everyone around them was telling them they were going to be great bodybuilders. In many cases they didn't have a clue what they were doing in the gym and were not eating properly to support muscle growth. But when you are genetically destined to look like a bodybuilder, that doesn't really matter. So although this is not pleasant to admit, chances are that if you have been training hard for ten years or more and don't yet look like the guys and gals in the magazines, you never will. Don't jump up and scream about how steroids are the answer, as we will get to that in just a minute.

What's Race Got To Do With It?

While all men may have been created equal in the eyes of God and the Declaration of Independence, we were not all equally gifted with favorable genetic attributes for bodybuilding. As any of you who follow the sport of bodybuilding know, black men currently dominate. If you look at the whole picture of who is bodybuilding in the gyms around America, it's mostly white men. So why would the small percentage of blacks involved have better physiques? I can't say that I have the definitive answer. At least in sports like basketball you can argue that culture has something to do with it, that playgrounds in every inner city are packed with young black kids feverishly working to improve their hoop skills so they can be the next multimillionaire NBA star with his own sneakers. In the case of bodybuilding, the advantage has to be that African-Americans seem to be born more often with the right bone structure, muscle insertions and shape, and small joints to develop a pro bodybuilder's type of physique. Some have speculated that 400 years of slavery had something to do with this. The men and women who were kidnapped from Africa and crammed into ships to cross the Atlantic often died on the arduous trip unless they were healthy and strong to begin with. Then, once they landed in the New World and were forced into hard physical labor from sunup to sundown, again only the hardiest men and women were able to survive. It is also said that slave owners practiced a disgusting brand of animal husbandry, allowing only the strongest and best workers among the men to 'breed,' while others were barbarically castrated. This is Darwin's evolution theory, the survival of the fittest, only accelerated to lightning speed. If all these assumptions are correct, the atrocities of slavery had the end result of creating a group of physically superior men and women.

This is not to say that there are not great bodybuilders of every race and ethnic group – there certainly are. There are merely general differences that often occur between them. For instance, there are plenty of huge guys competing at over 250 pounds these days. For some reason, most of the white guys this size have wider waists, thicker midsections, and bigger butts than their black peers who are the same size. Another generality is that Asian bodybuilders rarely are able to gain enough muscle mass to compete beyond the middleweight class, the limit of which is 176 pounds. This one is easy to figure out, as Asian men tend to be shorter and lighter-boned than either blacks or whites. But I have to stress again, there have been men and women of every race who have built fantastic physiques. One last thing you may have noticed is that Asian bodybuilders tend to have low calves, while most black athletes have high calves. Whites are all over the place. But since calves are really a minor factor in an overall physique package, it's merely an observation and nothing to worry about.

Can Genetics Be Changed?

I hate to be the bearer of bad news, but the simple truth is that genetics can't be changed. This means if you were meant to look like a pro bodybuilder, you will, and if you weren't, nothing is going to change that. Immediately many of you are thinking that massive doses of steroids do have that power to render meaningless any poor genetics you may have been dealt thanks to your parents. This is also untrue. Steroids certainly can make you much, much bigger than you were ever meant to be naturally, but even then you are limited. I have known plenty of guys who juiced their brains out and could never get past a certain point. Honestly, if steroids had this incredibly magic power, any of us could be as big as Ronnie Coleman or Markus Ruhl. Still, through tons of drugs, years of hard and heavy training, and enough food to feed a small nation, many guys do at least get to the approximate size of pro bodybuilders. That is to say, they may weigh 270 pounds and have 22-inch arms just like Jay Cutler. But they do not remotely look like Jay Cutler, because they don't have the same type of bone structure, muscle origins and insertions, small joints, and round muscle shape that he does. They are more often mistaken for wrestlers or NFL lineman than they are recognized as bodybuilders, particularly if they don't stay extremely lean.

To an extent, you can be smart about your training and add muscle to certain places to create an illusion, which is essentially what our sport is based on. For example, if you put a lot of mass on your shoulders and back without your waist getting any bigger, you will present the illusion of a smaller waist. Realize, however, that it will never be as impressive as when another person does the same thing that already has wider clavicles and narrower hips. You can also stress certain portions of your muscles, such as upper chest and outer thighs, to create a more aesthetically pleasing physique. But there will always be a few guys with absolutely perfect shape like Flex Wheeler, Danny Hester, or Dexter Jackson who look like a sculpted god no matter what exercises they choose.

So Fucking What?

This may sound disheartening. Why bother bodybuilding if you can't look like you belong on the Olympia stage? What a terrible way to look at it. That's like someone who loves golf deciding to quit playing because he will never be as good as Tiger Woods. Bodybuilding isn't really about the sport of bodybuilding. It's about the lifestyle, and about you making improvements and looking better than you ever had before. Even if you do compete, you are never in control of who will stand next to you and what they look like in comparison to you. All you can ever do is work on any weak points and try to make sure you present a better package every single time. And for most of you who will never compete, the main key is still self-improvement. If you started lifting weights weighing 100 pounds and now you're 150, that's awesome! Who gives a shit if Gunter Schlierkamp weighs twice as much? You can't compare yourself to others or else you are setting yourself up for failure – particularly if you choose to compare yourself to the genetic elite. Once you fully understand how very rare the genetic elite are in bodybuilding, you should never have to use their physiques as yardsticks to measure your own accomplishments.

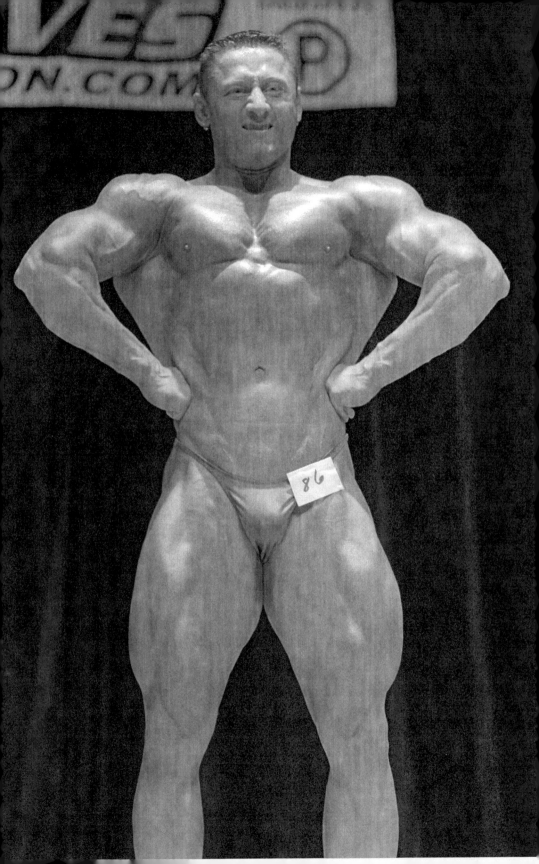

03

STEROIDS – THE TRUTH WILL SET YOU FREE

Steroids have grown to play an enormous role in bodybuilding in the 21st century, so there is understandably a lot of ground to cover. I'd like to start with clearing up a lot of the crap you have been spoon-fed by the media and the medical community for many years.

The scope of this book does not allow for a full technical discussion of all the various steroids and their use and abuse, and honestly, I am not qualified to address the issue to that depth and level of expertise. *Chemical Muscle Enhancement* by A. Rhea and *Anabolics 2008* by William Llewellyn are both excellent reference works that should be read by all before even considering their first cycle.

10 Big Fat Lies About Steroids – The Load Of Bullshit 'They' Want You To Believe

Few subjects are discussed regularly with such consistent lies and misinformation as anabolic/androgenic steroids (AAS). Those we trust to deliver honest information about important topics, such as television news shows, newspapers, magazines, and even our family doctors continue to perpetuate facts about steroids that are often completely inaccurate and sensationalized for dramatic effect. Whether they are intentionally trying to make a story sound more lurid as in the case of the mainstream media, or are attempting to scare us away from performance-enhancing drugs 'for our own good,' there is no excuse for lying. If something is really so bad as steroids are painted to be, then the true facts and evidence should be enough to deter us from using them. But as most of you already know, nearly everything you hear about steroids outside of bodybuilding magazines is a bunch of bullshit propaganda. Here are the ten big fat lies you hear most often about AAS, clearly exposed as the fictitious drivel they really are.

Big Fat Lie # 1:
Steroids Will Kill You!

I hear this one all the time, usually from some fat sack of shit two jelly donuts away from a heart attack, puffing away on a Marlboro. If steroids are so very deadly, shouldn't we have bodies piling up outside the hardcore gyms like stacks of firewood? In fact, can anyone name even one person who has died directly as a result of using steroids? The medical journals have discussed several such cases, but they were all very sick patients given large doses of oral steroids over extended periods of time who predictably enough, eventually developed major liver problems. Another study in Finland tried to say steroids led to early death by following a small group of powerlifters over roughly twenty years. Several of the premature deaths were actually suicides, and the others were related to other factors that may or may not have had any direct links to their past drug use. When you fire back with a retort like this, the fat sack of shit usually adopts a smug expression and utters the magic name that proves without a doubt steroids will kill you as surely as a 9 mm slug to the head – Lyle Alzado. The once-fearsome lineman went on a crusade in his dying days on television shows, convinced that his brain tumor was the result of his former steroid use. Aside from his own belief, there was never a shred of evidence to support his assertion. If we are to be objective for just a second, we all agree that occasionally people get brain tumors. It's tragic, but it happens. Given the sheer amount of people who use or have used steroids, it's completely feasible that one of these unfortunate cancer victims will have juiced at one time or another. This does not mean there is any more connection between the steroids and the tumor than there might be between his daily can of diet soda and the tumor. Bottom line, there is a dearth of evidence to back up this frequently repeated statement. I would never want to imply that steroids are harmless and do not have the potential for serious health problems when abused, but to portray them as being on the same level as cancer and heart disease as an epidemic is ludicrous.

Big Fat Lie # 2:
Steroid Users Are Cheating

Okay, whom are we supposedly cheating? Let's try to figure this out, shall we? In professional sports and even high-level amateur sports such as the Olympic games, there is drug testing. This does not stop nearly all of these athletes from using steroids by a long shot They all just beat the test one way or another because they know everyone else does too. So if everyone is 'cheating' in high-level sports, then in reality no one is cheating. The only legitimate example I can think of where a steroid user is cheating is when he or she enters a drug-tested bodybuilding or powerlifting competition and passes him or herself off as being drug-free in order to gain an unfair advantage. These pathetic jerk-offs are truly morally bankrupt, so I have no problem in labeling them as cheaters. In non-tested events, drug use is tacitly permitted, so choosing to compete in them naturally is something done at the athlete's own discretion, knowing that they are at a distinct disadvantage. Yet the vast majority of steroid users are recreational or cosmetic bodybuilders who will never enter a contest of any sort. He or she uses drugs as an adjunct to a disciplined training and eating regimen purely to improve the appearance. Who are these guys and gals cheating by doing so? The skinny guy with the love handles at Bally's who complains that he can't get any results from the gym when he trains like a pussy (missing workouts all the time, to boot) and eats a bunch of garbage? Get real. Steroid users aren't cheating anyone, so shut up with that nonsense. If we are cheating anyone, it's Mother Nature, and she can be a bitch anyway.

Big Fat Lie # 3:
Steroid Users Are Lazy

Are there some steroid users who use the drugs as a crutch and don't work all that hard in the gym or eat the best diet? Sure there are, but they are definitely in the minority. Most steroid users, and I have personally known hundreds over the years, are far more devoted to their training and nutrition than the average gym denizen. They tend to read constantly in search of the latest information on exercise, nutrition, supplements, and yes, drugs as well. You will see them training with 100% intensity, never missing workouts or meals, totally dedicated and disciplined. Most of them have been living this demanding lifestyle for many years, yet as soon as someone finds out they also happen to use steroids, all that hard work is instantly dismissed or ignored. The average knucklehead who does nothing but screw around with bench presses in horrible form and eats fast food all day can now feel superior to the 'juicer,' who didn't really work for that incredible body. Little do they know that many of these anabolic gods and goddesses looked great long before they even took their first pill or injection, because they had already been training and eating right for a few years. I find it hilarious that the ones who like to label steroid users as lazy are the same ones who are too lazy to learn how to train right and won't make any effort to prepare and eat five to eight nutritious meals every day.

Big Fat Lie # 4:
Juice Will Have You Looking Like Jay Cutler In A Week

There is the belief among many that all one needs to do is start to use steroids, and in a short time, they will resemble freaks like Jay Cutler, Lee Priest, and Chris Cormier. I can almost excuse the general public for buying into this horseshit, because they are usually ignorant about such matters. Worse is when natural bodybuilders say it – and I hate to admit I used to do this a few years ago too. I have actually overheard natural guys who weigh no more than 160 pounds at 5-9 say something like, "yeah, if I used steroids I would be just as big as that Ronnie Coleman." The fuck you would, idiot. Ronnie Coleman turned professional back in 1991 when he was still natural, and he was already competing at 215 with arms over twenty inches. Jay Cutler weighed a husky 180 pounds at 5-9 when he started training, and just a year later he was tipping the scales at over 240 pounds. Don't these guys get it? Some people are meant to be huge and others just aren't. It takes three things to look like an IFBB pro: years of hard training and good nutrition, extremely rare genetics, and finally drugs. The drugs are obviously a big part of the look, but the least significant of the three factors. You can train hard and eat right for twenty years and take all the drugs in existence, but without the right genetics you will never, ever look like Jay or Ronnie. Seriously, do you think you could take lanky Leonardo DiCaprio, ship him out to Gold's Venice to train with Charles Glass, put him on a pro-level stack of 'roids and GH, and he would ever be able to stand next to the likes of Levrone and Gunter? Sorry to ruin your delusion, but no frigging way. If you honestly believe the only difference between the pro's and the garden-variety wannabe bodybuilders at your gym is steroids, you are sadly mistaken.

Big Fat Lie # 5:
All Gains From 'Roids Disappear When You Go Off

Another whopper, this one. I have watched many a bodybuilder go off steroids, and the only ones who lost everything they gained from their cycles were those who quit training entirely. I have seen some maintain as much as 80% of the gains they made from steroids, while the average seems to be closer to 40-50%. You also need to realize that there is a cumulative effect for most bodybuilders who will do anywhere from ten to fifty 6-15 week cycles before quitting for good. Hypothetically, let's say a man starts juicing at the age of twenty-two, weighing 170 pounds. Twelve years and thirty cycles later, his weight is up to 270 pounds. This is by no means a farfetched transformation, as many thousands have made similar progress. At age thirty-four, he decides he has had a good run with anabolics, but no longer wishes to use them. He continues to train hard and heavy (though probably not as heavy), and eats plenty of good food and supplements. Is our imaginary man going to shrivel down to 170 now? Not a chance. He may drop from 270 down to 240 or 230, and fifteen pounds of such a loss could easily be water retention from the more androgenic compounds like test or d-bol. He is still going to be a very big, strong man, and certainly much more so than if he had never used steroids. It is no secret that many of the most thickly-developed natural bodybuilders are the guys who used to use steroids in the past. There is no way all the additional muscle mass is going to magically evaporate once you stop using gear unless you magically quit workout out.

Big Fat Lie # 6:
Steroid Users Are Lowlifes And Criminals

There is a stereotype of the average steroid user as being some thug named Vinny who sells recreational drugs, beats his girlfriend, and works as a mob enforcer. I think we get this from the movies and TV, since most juiced-up guys working in Hollywood are only able to land bit parts as thugs and gangsters. I am sure there are a few guys who fit this seedy mold, but at least 90% of all steroid users are otherwise respectable, law-abiding citizens. If you have not yet read Rick Collins' book Legal Muscle (available online at www.SteroidLaw.com) you owe it to yourself to get a copy and read it as soon as you can. Rick is a criminal defense attorney who has represented more men and women charged with steroid possession than any other lawyer in history. And he will tell you that nearly all of his clients have good jobs and families, are productive members of society, and a threat to no one. Unfortunately, the laws are such that if such a 'good guy' is caught with steroids in his possession, he is lumped into the same category as heroin addicts and crack dealers. In fact, due to the ignorance of law enforcement agencies regarding the quantities of drugs we bodybuilders use, many unlucky souls are charged with distribution and face far stiffer penalties under the legal system. Rick goes into all this with a great deal more detail, insight, and eloquence than I possibly could, but suffice to say that his book thoroughly trashes the stereotype of who steroid users really are.

Big Fat Lie # 7:
Steroids Kill Your Sex Drive And Make You Impotent

Anyone who would fall for this lie has obviously never used steroids or they would laugh as loud as I do when I hear it. The effect steroids have on your sex drive and performance ability is nothing short of amazing. On a good cycle including a gram or two of testosterone a week, a man in his thirties or forties has the sexual capabilities he had at eighteen – only hopefully now he doesn't come after ten seconds of thrusting! When you're juiced, you think about sex every waking moment, and often even all your dreams involve sexual encounters. You have steel-like erections many times a day with even the slightest bit of visual or tactile stimulation. And can you hit that coochie? Good God, if you had a houseful of ten hot women you could probably do them all once a day, and do them very well I might add (Steve Blechman, I would be willing to test out this theory if you could set it up – all in the name of science!). You may find yourself being a little rougher with your woman during the act because you are so damned horny. Add the powerful hips you developed from heavy squatting and deadlifting into the equation, and you could penetrate a brick wall if you had to. In many ways steroids can turn a man with a normal sexual appetite and performance abilities into a virtual porn star. You can get it up and keep it up like few mortal men can. The only problem is that it is not always possible for a man in this situation to have a woman with an equal appetite for lovin'. Of course, once you go off the steroids, there will be a temporary period of a month to three months where your libido will crash and erections may be a problem. This almost always amends itself once your body begins producing adequate testosterone on its own once again. And none of ever has to worry about erections ever again anyway, the greedy pharmaceutical industry had made sure of that.

Big Fat Lie # 8:
Steroids Will Turn You Into A Violent Asshole

Steroids can increase feelings of aggression and make it harder to control your temper. So if a man already has a problem with being hostile and violent, it's likely that steroids can exacerbate this. But again, going back to my own anecdotal evidence culled from years of observation, the only guys I ever knew who were assholes on juice were assholes long before they started using. I have never seen an even-tempered person suddenly transform into a raging maniac from steroids. Very young guys seem to be the most prone to violent or aggressive behavior while on steroids, but then again the same can be said about many young, immature guys who have never been near a steroid. Come on now, do you think all the gangbangers running around shooting up the 'hood and beating down rivals are on Sustanon and Deca? The reality is that most steroid users I know tend to actually be less hostile and unpleasant than the average person. Most of us know how to apply all that aggression toward our training, where it has a beneficial result.

Big Fat Lie # 9:
Steroids Are Destroying American's Youth!

I do not condone steroid use by teenagers. At the same time, I think it has been wildly exaggerated as to how many high-school students are into steroids. I have seen statistics as low as 3% and as high as 20%. That's a pretty big range, which makes it tough to believe we even have anything like an accurate idea of what the percentage really is. But that's not really important. If I was a parent, and I do happen to have a son and a daughter myself, I would be far more concerned with Junior drinking alcohol, smoking marijuana, taking Ecstasy, or snorting cocaine. I watch the news and read the papers, and I never seem to read about fatal car accidents or drug overdoses involving teenagers and steroids. Nobody is slipping a couple tablets of Winstrol into a 16-year-old girl's drink and committing a date rape. Teens have no business using steroids, but as far as being a threat, there are about a hundred other drugs far worse to worry about. Any time you hear differently you can be sure it's a slow news day down at Channel Five.

Big Fat Lie # 10:
You Can Get Just As Big With Supplements

Some supplements will give you noticeable results, but to insinuate for even a second that you can build the same exact physique using only legal supplements is silly. I know it's tempting to look at the ads with the before and after pictures and start thinking the product being sold is actually 100% responsible for all the rapid muscle gain and fat loss you see, but it's just not possible to duplicate the effects of powerful drugs without using them. Maybe in the distant future supplements will reach that point of effectiveness, but we are nowhere near that point at present.

Those are the top ten big fat lies being floated around concerning steroids. You have probably heard most of them and perhaps even bought into one or more of them, but by now you should be able to see the massive campaign of ignorance and misinformation that the media and medical industry has been feeding us. To them I say, the truth will set you free, and if the truth about steroids were as awful as they make it out to be, I would not hesitate to stand out against them. But because most of what we hear about steroids is untrue or wildly exaggerated, I can't take that stand. Think for yourself and form your own opinions based only on the facts, and you can't go wrong.

Are You Ready To Juice?

Let's suppose you have made your decision as a responsible adult based on the facts. You think you're ready to take the big plunge. You've decided that your life just won't be complete unless you resemble the huge, veiny, freaks you see on the pages of the muscle magazines. And you're no dummy – you realize that this inhuman look simply isn't possible without some serious pharmaceutical assistance. You want to start using steroids and join the ranks of the truly big boys, leaving the world of the physically average light years behind. Though steroids are against the law, that's not going to deter you from your dream. But before you make your initial buy and begin your virgin cycle, you'd better be ready. I'm sure you think you already are. Maybe so, Sparky, and maybe not. Ask yourself these questions before making this very important decision that will have a significant impact on your life.

How Old Are You?

When it comes to issues like voting, driving a motor vehicle, or buying alcohol, we have clear-cut demarcations made by lawmakers that tell us what age one should be. There is no such age that anyone can say is appropriate for using steroids. The two areas in question are the physical and mental maturity of the individual. Some boys have completed adolescence by age fifteen, meaning that they have reached their full adult height, their voices have changed, and they exhibit other signs of developmental maturity such as facial hair. Another fifteen-year-old may have barely started puberty and still resemble a child. My feeling is that no one should think of using steroids until they have at least completed this easily discernable process. Mental/emotional maturity is a bit more difficult to measure. Some 18-year-olds are mature and responsible, while others can be even older and yet still think and act like children in many ways. A child should not be introducing substances into their body that will be drastically altering their hormonal profile and their muscle mass. They will have a very hard time dealing with these changes. It's a tough call, and I doubt that many immature young men have the ability to objectively evaluate this. I can state with confidence that no one under the age of 18 should be using anabolics. As a writer and the owner of a bodybuilding web site, I often get e-mails asking for advice regarding steroids from boys as young as thirteen years old. They are never happy when I respond with my blunt sentiments, but I will not be a part of someone using steroids so prematurely. Steroids aren't for kids, bottom line.

How Serious Are You About Bodybuilding?

Is lifting just a hobby for you, something you do on and off? Steroids are powerful drugs, and I consider them to be tools that dedicated men and women use to enhance the results from intense training and solid nutrition. If you are just a dabbler who only trains when summer's coming or to pump up your arms a little bit, then don't waste your time and money on steroids. You won't see very good results anyway with that half-ass attitude, even on a good test/d-bol/deca cycle. Don't bother going to the trouble of getting and using ergogenic drugs if you aren't totally committed to becoming bigger and stronger than 99% of the guys at the gym who are there spinning their wheels and chit-chatting about last night's football game. You'd better be someone who trains hard, and is always trying to push his intensity with the weights even higher. These drugs are meant for those who consider themselves athletes, and who will devote ten to fifteen-week blocks of time for their cycles to push harder than ever before at the gym and support it all with top-quality food and supplements. If you're just gonna screw around and train when you feel like it and eat when and what you fancy, forget it. You're unworthy of the benefits that steroids impart.

Do You Know How To Train?

A lot of guys, especially young guys, jump the gun and get on a cycle before they even have a basic handle on training. I have seen tons of these kids who make such ignorant mistakes as training only a couple bodyparts (usually arms and chest), training the same muscle groups every day, and not even knowing which exercises work what muscles. Just the other day a kid with the tell-tale red, puffy 'roid face on an otherwise lean body saw me doing barbell rows and asked me what they were for. When I told him rows built your lats, he nodded and looked away. He had just lost interest because back was something he didn't even train. A lot of guys know which exercises to do and follow a decent split routine, but their form just sucks sweaty ass. They heave and throw the weights around as if every exercise was meant to work the entire body. They use far too much weight and rely on spotters to lift half of it for them, or else they use only a fraction of the full range of motion. I think we've all seen the guys who load up the leg press with half a ton or more and proceed to do two-inch reps. If any of this sounds eerily familiar, you're not ready to use steroids yet. With all the information on proper training available these days in magazines, books, on the Internet, and on videos, you have no excuse to be so ignorant. Only when you have mastered the fine art of weight training should you consider adding steroids to your regimen.

Do You Know How To Eat?

Without the right nutritional support, all the steroids in the world will not allow you to reach your goals. Many users get on their first cycle planning on gaining twenty or thirty pounds of muscle in a couple months. Much to their consternation, they often fall far short of these goals. What they fail to realize is that you still need to eat 5-7 times a day, increasing both protein and caloric intake, for the steroids to do their job and synthesize new muscle tissue. If you continue to eat three square meals a day (or fewer) like the untrained general public and consume anything less than 1.5 grams of protein per pound of bodyweight a day, you won't be a whole hell of a lot bigger when the cycle is over. Eating like a bodybuilder does is a job. You stick to a rigid schedule of eating every two hours, never missing a meal. High-quality protein is the first priority, so every day you put down a shitload of red meat, chicken, eggs, fish, and protein shakes and bars. Yet you also need sufficient carbohydrates and healthy fats to support training and recovery. While a very gifted minority can get away with missing meals and eating mostly junk, for most lifters this poor nutritional plan would result in very dismal gains. Other guys start using steroids to "cut up" or "get ripped," thinking that the drugs will do all the work while they can continue to eat as they always do. Sorry to break it to you, but unless you diet strictly and do plenty of cardio, all the Winstrol and Primobolan in the world won't give you a six-pack of abs and striated delts. If you don't have much knowledge on proper nutrition and supplementation, you'd better get some before you entertain the notion of getting on some gear.

Have You Built A Natural Base?

Training naturally for a few years before using steroids is highly recommended for two key reasons. First, you need this time to learn proper form and develop a mind-muscle connection. There is a world of difference between going through the motions of any exercise and actually training the muscle hard. A lot of this has to do with neural learning, and simply can't be rushed. For instance, it often takes a few years for many trainers to feel their lats working, or to learn how to make squats work more quads and less glutes and lower back. The second reason has to do with safety. Steroids have the power to allow your muscle size and strength to increase very rapidly in a short time. Great, right? Not always. We need to remember that our muscles are attached to our bodies with tendons. Unlike muscles, tendons do not have a great deal of potential for growth. Over years of regular training with heavy weights, they will become thicker, but they have nowhere near the potential for growth as muscle tissue does. Many steroid users experience muscle tears for this very reason. A man may go from 180 to 240 pounds after a few cycles, and his bench press might shoot up from 275 pounds to over 450 pounds. Certainly his chest will be much thicker and fuller. However, the tendons that connect those newly-huge pecs to his skeleton are not. Put them under a strain too much for them to bear enough times, and sooner or later something has to give. Because the tendons have a poor blood supply, they are also very slow to heal. By taking a few years and becoming very strong without steroids, you build your tendons up and at least minimize the chance of this scenario happening to you.

Do You Think Being Big Will Solve All Your Problems?

A lot of us begin bodybuilding in hopes of resolving issues of insecurity, inadequacy, and insignificance. I know that was what drove me to pick up my first weights as a 95-pound high school freshman back in the day. The belief (and this is by no means limited to adolescents) is that if they can become big and muscular, they will earn instant respect and inspire fear from their fellow males, and the hot chicks that laugh at them now will be begging for the privilege of being boinked. In essence, they see steroids as the quick fix to all their problems in life. Take it from someone who has built the body he dreamed of as a teenager and knows plenty of others who also have – you're still the same person inside when it's all said and done. You may have more confidence, but extra muscle mass does nothing to improve your actual personality and ability to relate to other people. Deep-rooted emotional issues don't magically disappear when you change your appearance. And you may not believe this, but very few women actually find the "steroid look" attractive. Most women are repulsed and/or intimidated by all that bulk. Muscles will not help you gain instant acceptance in society, either. Usually very large bodybuilders are treated as freaks in the negative connotation of the word and stereotyped as stupid and narcissistic. Become big because you want to for your own satisfaction, not because you think huge muscles will be your ticket to a charmed life. No drug can do that for you.

Can You Afford Steroids?

Before you get wrapped up in the life of a juicer, you need to have access to some disposable income. Steroids are not cheap like they were in the 70's and 80's. Even a modest eight-week cycle of cheapo Mexican test and deca will set you back about a grand. Should you decide to use human-grade gear and add in items like growth hormone, a cycle can run well over two or three grand. Most juicers do two to four cycles a year, so do the math. If you're a struggling student or otherwise barely making ends meet, you're not ready to use steroids yet. What good are 'roids if you can't afford the right food and supplements, or you have to take the bus to the gym? And if you have dependents like a wife and young kids, don't even dream of buying steroids unless you have plenty of money left over for your family's needs. Anyone who deprives their family just so they can put a few pounds of muscle on is a first-class jackass in my book. And know this – almost nobody does just one cycle. As soon as your drugs run out and you start losing that jacked-up body, you're gonna want to get more right away. If you can't buy more because you're too broke, it's gonna suck to be you.

Have You Researched The Subject?

Pay special attention to this question, because it's a common area where steroid users fuck up. Steroids are not as deadly as the media has duped Americans into thinking they are, but they are by no means harmless. Used incorrectly and without certain ancillary drugs, the results can be disastrous. You need to know what the various drugs are, what their potential dangers and side effects are, and what you may need to take along with them to prevent these problems. You also have to have a good idea what constitutes reasonable dosages. Use too little and all that will happen is a lack of results. Use too much, or too much of the more dangerous items, and you can expect liver damage, gyno, hair loss, and acne so bad it would make an Oxy-clean pad run away screaming. For instance, many novice users are unaware that taking oral versions of steroids is very tough on the liver, and will pop endless tabs of D-bol and Anadrol for months on end. Maybe they're afraid of needles, or just too lazy to go to the trouble of loading up syringes and injecting when they can just throw a pill down the hatch. Other guys will use extremely androgenic compounds like test or Anadrol without some sort of estrogen blocker or aromatase inhibitor like Nolvadex, Arimidex, or Clomid and wonder why their nipples swell up into painful little man-tits. If your hairline is already receding or thinning, you'd better include Proscar/finasteride in your cycle unless you want a cue-ball head. With all the steroid reference books and the info on so many web sites as available resources, the only reason a steroid user today would make these mistakes is out of sheer laziness. I say if you can't even take the time and make the effort to become educated about these drugs, you certainly have no right to use them. It's just my opinion, but I happen to be correct.

Can You Keep Your Mouth Shut?

Steroids, as we all know, are against the law. Luckily for those who choose to buy and use them, law enforcement authorities are usually far too concerned with recreational drugs like cocaine, heroin, methamphetamines, and Ecstasy to harass the dudes walking around with 21-inch arms about what might be in their medicine cabinets. After all, more than a few cops use steroids themselves. As long as you're discreet and keep your steroid use to yourself, you will probably never have a problem. If instead you shoot your mouth off all the time about your cycles and what you've used or plan to use, you might start turning the odds against you. Police officers, DEA agents, and Customs officials aren't always in uniform, you know. They could be the guy spotting you on squats who you brag to about how you just smuggled a ton of gear in over the Mexican border. They could be the buff bouncer at the nightclub you share all your cycle details with. They might even be the person in the online chat room who offers to sell you a few bottles of tren. If you use steroids, however obvious that fact may be, you need to keep a low profile about it unless you just have to know what it's like to be arrested and see the inside of a jail cell.

Are You An Asshole?

Steroids don't turn guys into assholes, but if you're already one to start with, they can easily make you someone so despicable that a lot of people will wish you were dead. Do you start fights over someone looking at you the wrong way? Do you succumb to road rage and become a time bomb on four wheels? Do you have a history of verbal and/or physical abuse toward the ones you love? Is your temper already on a short fuse? If you answered yes to any of these, stay the hell away from steroids. Heightened aggression is a very common side effect of steroids, but most users have the ability to keep it all under control. A few jerks can't, and they usually end up assaulting someone when they flip out. Combined with the superhuman size and strength of many juicers, this can occasionally even end in someone dying. It's just bad, bad news for the asshole and anyone unfortunate enough to be around them. Do the world a favor if you fit this description and stay off 'roids. In fact, take an anger management class and get on some sedatives while you're at it. Angry people suck!

Are You Prepared To Cycle Off?

Don't get involved in this thinking you'll be on a constant cycle for the rest of your life. Sure, you can do that, but don't expect to live past forty or fifty at most. Your body needs regular breaks off the gear to let your organs regenerate and your own natural hormones to start being produced again. Understand that you will lose a percentage of your "assisted" size and strength during these clean-out periods, often very rapidly. Your sex drive and ability to sustain an erection may also be severely impacted at this time. Many juicers experience deep depression as a result, and it's not uncommon for them to either quit training altogether while they're clean, or never really go off. The practice of "bridging" heavy cycles with lighter cycles of Winstrol or Primobolan just means you've changed your stack. You're still on steroids. You need to realize that it's very important to give your body a break from the drugs, no matter how tough it is to lose your superhuman status for a time. If you can't deal with that inevitability, you're better off never even using steroids.

What do you say now? Hopefully if you are thinking about using steroids these questions made you reflect on whether or not it's the right decision for you, at this time or ever. In the end the choice is totally yours, but be smart and choose wisely.

The Most Popular Drugs And How They Are Used

As I said at the beginning of this chapter, there are those far more qualified than I to give full discourses on steroids, getting into the actual chemistry of them, and breaking down complex cycles to follow. What I can offer is a general overview from someone in the trenches. The most popular drugs have always been the ones that are cheapest and most readily available. Various esters and blends of testosterone have been a staple in the training regimen of many a lifter for decades, and most consider it the base around which they build their cycles. Test is almost always injected. The other superstar of the steroid world is nandrolone decanoate, otherwise known as deca. The humble cycle of testosterone and deca has probably put more muscle on more human beings than any other. Doses for each range from 300 milligrams a week all the way up to one or two thousand. Oral steroids are also frequently added in, the two most popular being methandrostenolone (D-bol) and oxymetholone (Anadrol 50). There are also several other highly used steroids, including trenbolone, boldenone (Equipoise), stanozolol (Winstrol), methenolone (Primobolan), and oxandrolone (Anavar). These days, it is common practice for bodybuilders to stack one or two of the more 'androgenic' agents such as test and d-bol with one or two products more toward the 'anabolic' end of the spectrum such as deca, Equipoise, or Winstrol. Weekly milligram totals can range from a very conservative five or six hundred milligrams all the way to a more kamikaze approach of three to ten thousand milligrams. There are also other drugs involved, such as Human Growth Hormone (GH), insulin, and IGF-1. To prevent excess estrogen conversion, which can result in bitch tits or gynocemastia, drugs such as Nolvadex, Clomid, or Arimidex are used. For fat-burning purposes, many bodybuilders employ one or more of the following: clenbuterol, thyroid hormone, and DNP. When the cycle is over, Clomid and HCG are usually administered in an effort to jump-start the body's own testosterone production. Otherwise, the dreaded 'crash' occurs, where the enhanced size, strength, and sex drive that comes while using the drugs all fades away quickly. Whole books have been written about steroids, and I encourage you to read several so that you are well-informed enough to make the right decisions and stay as healthy as possible.

My Life On The Dark Side

The following is an interview I did with myself on the web site www.testosterone.net in 2001, where I was both the interviewer and the subject. It appeared online several years ago, and details my own experiences with steroids. Until now I have been too ashamed to even admit in print that I have used steroids.

Underground Tap
The Natural Man who Switched Colors

By Ron Harris

Why would someone who once vehemently rallied the industry against steroids eventually succumb to their call? Why would a man who was proud to be 100 % drug-free for life give up this hallowed status? "Joe Natural" appeared in magazines throughout the 1990's and was one of a handful of well-known natural bodybuilders who did their best to convince magazine readers that steroids were deadly, and that using them branded you as a lazy cheater. Somewhere along the way he slipped off the 'righteous' path, and began to use steroids. Why did he do it? What did he discover about using steroids? Does he harbor any regrets? What would he say to his fans and natural bodybuilders now? These were a few of the answers I was looking for when I sat down to talk to a man who betrayed his former ideals.

Let's kick this right off with the brutal questions. How could you use steroids after being such a crusader for years?

It definitely wasn't an easy decision. As you said, a lot of natural guys looked up to me for getting the anti-drug message out there, and I took a lot of pride in being natural. Maybe I took too much pride. A lot of the pro's and amateurs who were 'enhanced' didn't take kindly to my holier-than-thou attitude. Some of them teased me about it. I knew that once I took that first pill or shot, I would be letting down a lot of people and setting myself up to be lambasted as a hypocrite. But at that point, it was a little over four years ago, I had pretty much hit the genetic ceiling. I had been training naturally for twelve years, and new gains were so few and far between that training was starting to lose its luster for me. Another influencing factor was that I had watched a lot of guys on drugs over the years around me, and I had yet to see one drop dead or needing a new liver. It became clear that steroids were not as dangerous as I had believed, and that I had been blowing the dangers out of proportion while warning people. I was really talking out of my ass, just repeating a lot of what I had read and heard. And not that I had any plans of entering the Mr. Olympia, but I felt there was still a lot more I wanted to do with my physique in terms of size and shape. If I stayed natural, most of that would never be realized. That's not defeatist, that's just how it is.

What was your first cycle?

Let me preface all the dosage stuff by saying that I've never used extreme amounts of anabolics. If any of your readers are hoping for something out of 'The Dead Pool," they're not going to get it from me. I do believe that the risks involved with steroids are amplified when you use grams and grams of gear a week. That's one. Two, I have a family, and I could never justify spending a ton of money when I could be spoiling my wife and kids instead. For instance, I would never buy GH or something that expensive. A couple cycles of that and you could've taken your family to the

Bahamas for a week. Three, I'm not trying to weigh 300 pounds. Nothing against those guys who do. That's their prerogative, and if they want to compete in the big shows, they have no choice but to use anything and everything. I admire a lot of those physiques, but the reality is that without the right genetics few of us could ever look like them, even with the very best drugs and training.

My first cycle was a single Sustanon-250 a week, plus 300 or 400 mg. of Norandren, one of the Mexican vet decas, for eight weeks. Nothing major, but I got bigger and stronger. I think my weight only went up ten pounds, but it looked like twenty. My strength started getting ridiculous. I finally got that really full look to the muscles that I had never had.

Who knew you were using at that point?

Aside from me and my wife, it's tough to say. Nobody ever came up and said anything to my face except for snide, veiled remarks. I'm sure a lot of people at my gym knew. I had always been able to tell when guys were on or off stuff, so I probably wasn't fooling too many people.

How long did you wait before you went on again?

Not long at all. In fact, that first year I was a little over-eager. I did something like five different cycles of 6-10 weeks. I was probably on about ¾ of the time or more.

What other kinds of drugs did you try?

I went with what was relatively cheap and available. I tried various types of test with different vet decas, usually about 500 grams of each a week. Those always seemed to work well, but using those 50 mg. per ml. vet decas means you have to put a lot of damned oil in your ass. At one point I did a cycle that was nothing but 1000 mg. of Steris cypionate a week, because I had read that you might as well just use a lot of test instead of stacking. One thing I got out of that year was to stay away from test. For me, it caused too much acne and water retention. That cypionate stack was the last one I did for two years.

Why did you stop again?

I was getting frustrated with getting so big and strong, then losing it all when I came off. Plus my gut was getting bigger, and I was looking older when I was on. My wife didn't even want to touch my back anymore, it disgusted her so much. After nearly a solid year of being on, I cleaned out again.

Surely after all that time, everybody must have known you weren't natural anymore.

I would imagine so. It's one of those things where everyone talks behind your back. Only a few people had the nerve to come out and ask me, although some of them did it without any tact.

What was your comeback?

If there were other people around, I would brush them off without answering. A question posed that rudely doesn't deserve the dignity of an answer. If we were alone or a group of people wasn't hovering around, I would explain that yes, I had tried some anabolics. I certainly was never proud of it. Some of my friends who were natural were disappointed, but they didn't pass judgement – at least not to my face. I felt pretty bad about them. One guy who is the president of a natural organization I used to compete in saw a picture of me in a magazine with the new size and never talked to me again. That hurt, because he was one of my mentors in the very beginning when I was just a confused little teenager looking for direction. Another time I showed up at a well-known physique photographer's studio for a photo shoot, and he immediately knew. I was 20 pounds heavier than the last time he had shot me two years before. That was when I was using all that test, and the acne on my back was a dead giveaway. I felt bad that he knew, but he wasn't too shocked. He had seen his fair share of natural guys who had gone the other way. I think he made some joke about how great my training must be going lately.

What happened after the two years that made you start up again?

Basically in that time I had read up a lot more and saw that I had been doing some things wrong. I did a cycle of Reforvit-B and Equipose while I was dieting for some photo shoots and a series of TV commercials I had been cast in. To my surprise, I didn't get any acne, or hold any water. I also was able to hold onto a bit more of the size than I ever had before. A few months later I tried D-bol tabs and Deca, and came away from that cycle with a little bit more mass. My shape was getting better as well. Most recently I did another cycle of D-bol and Deca, and finally did the Clomid and HCG at the end. What a difference! Instead of losing 85 % of what I had gained, I only lost maybe 50 %. Three steps forward and two steps back still puts you ahead of where you started from.

What do you have to say to other natural guys who might be pondering the same decision about trying?

It all comes down to what you want to look like, and whether you're willing to take a little risk to get there. For instance, there are some natural guys who would be morons to start using steroids. Tito Raymond is a good example. He looks incredible clean, and even manages to make the top three in non-tested national shows. Why would he ever need to use drugs? Then again, with him and others like Skip LaCour, you're talking about genetic freaks. Some guys just luck out with tiny joints and long, full muscle bellies. They can look awesome even at fairly light bodyweights. Once in a while you get guys like Skip who can be just as big or bigger than most guys on drugs. If I could have looked like them naturally, I would never have popped that 'roid cherry. Most of us can never be that impressive without a little help. Then again, it takes at least five to ten years of heavy training and good nutrition before you have any idea what your genetic potential really is. Most guys on drugs never tried to take their bodies to the ultimate level that they could naturally.

So you're still moralizing, now it's against other guys on drugs?

That's not exactly it. I'm saying that if you are going to use steroids, you should at least have learned how to train and eat properly and built some kind of solid base. I've seen little 100-pound brats walk into the gym for the first time looking for a dealer. That just pisses me off. To me that's like trying to drive a tank without even knowing how to drive a car. You're trying to jump way ahead of where you should be at that stage.

Now that you've done all these cycles, are you planning to compete again? And will it be in a natural show?

I haven't in years, but I'm sure I will again. I really have two options. I could load up and do a non-tested show, but I wouldn't be able to win anything above the local level unless I had some dumb luck and didn't have any genetic superiors to face. I look good on drugs, but there are a lot of guys who look better in terms of size and shape. I'm 5-9, and I would be about 205 pounds with all those nasty striations. Guys my height at the NPC Nationals average 220-240 pounds. If I did one of the natural shows where you have to be clean for a year, like Team Universe or Musclemania, I could do pretty well. But I attribute that to the drugs. If I had never done any, I wouldn't have a chance against these black guys with the 19-inch arms and 25-inch waists that dominate the natural shows. It probably sounds racist, but I think a lot of white guys need to have some cycles behind them to be able to compete against black guys on a fair level in natural contests. I actually think the non-tested shows are more fair to non-blacks. The drugs help even out the playing field.

How many of those guys in natural shows do you think are really clean?

I think nearly all of them are clean, as interpreted by the rules of that particular organization. On the East Coast, there's the ANBC, where everyone needs to be drug-free for life to compete (*note: now defunct*). Then you have the NPC natural shows, where it's always one year. You have guys like Todd Smith, who used to be a big 260-pound freak, coming into shows like the Ironman Naturally at 220 and kicking ass over the guys who never took anything. But you can't fault Todd for it. He's following the rules as they stand. There are a few guys who will try to sneak through while on drugs. I consider them lower than dog shit.

What would you say the best and worst things about steroids are, from your experience?

The best thing is definitely the fact that when you're on, you know with absolute certainty that if you train your ass off, you will make gains. When I was clean all those years, I would do everything right with training, eating, and rest, and still there would be long stretches where I wouldn't gain an ounce. It gives you so much more confidence to train brutally hard when you know there will be a payoff. You can't wait for your next workout. Another thing is that you don't have to worry about overtraining as much. A few extra sets when you're on gear won't hurt your progress, it probably helps. The worst things are for me, not being able to hold that nice full look without the drugs and losing some of that crazy strength. Another hassle is getting the drugs. I've had experiences where I was burned with fake crap, frightening moments smuggling stuff in across the border, and long delays in ordering through the mail. I've never particularly liked the shots, either. My wife has to do them for me, and she's usually less than thrilled to help out.

Are you concerned about your health?

Maybe a tad, but it doesn't keep me up at night. The cycles I do these days don't even add up to a gram a week, and I stay away from the really toxic stuff like Anadrol. Plus I take plenty of time off, sometimes up to six months between cycles, but always at least two months. I'm just trying to add about five pounds of permanent quality muscle a year. I'm sure a lot of readers who aspire to be 300 pounds will laugh at that, but five pounds is a big difference when you've been training for sixteen years. Without the drugs, it might take me three or four years to get those five pounds at this point. The longer you've been training and the closer you get to your genetic potential, the harder it is to make any further gains.

What about morals? Do you feel guilty about using steroids when you had been a role model for a lot of young natural bodybuilders?

Like I said, I do feel bad if some guys wanted me to stay clean, but a lot of that is the "us versus them" mentality that many natural guys have. The disdain they feel for bodybuilders who choose to use anabolics borders on hate. I confess that I used to be like that. If someone was on drugs, they were a bad person, and I was morally superior to them. Over the years I saw how ridiculous that was. Sure, steroids are illegal, but so are a lot of things people do. I know some natural bodybuilders who smoke pot on a regular basis, yet they still sneer at those "frigging juicehead assholes." Legally, anyone can walk into a liquor store and buy a half-gallon of vodka and a carton of cigarettes, both of which kill millions of Americans every year. But if a dedicated athlete wants to take something in reasonable doses to enhance his physique and performance, he's a bad guy. To me that's ludicrous.

If you could do it all over again, would you have gone on drugs earlier?

I don't think so. All those years of training naturally taught me a lot about my body and how to train and eat for the best results. If I had started in my early twenties, like a lot of guys, I would never have reached the level of expertise that I have now. I wouldn't have had to. Another thing is that I like to say that I built the majority of my physique without any drugs. I give the 'roids credit for the last 15 % or so. Sometimes I wonder where I'd be if I had never taken the plunge four years ago. All I would really have is the pride of having accomplished whatever I would have naturally, and I feel like that pride was a bit overblown and pompous anyway.

Now that you've been on both sides, what would you like to say to the two camps?

For the natural guys, they need to get off the moral high horse. Nobody is keeping them from using drugs. It's a decision they made, so they shouldn't fault someone else for making a different choice. They also need to get the bullshit idea out of their heads that guys on drugs don't work hard. The majority of guys on drugs, especially when you're talking about guys who compete, work their asses off. With the help of the chemicals, they just get much better results. Bodybuilders on drugs aren't the enemy. They are comrades who do something different. For the guys who use drugs, they should give a lot of respect to natural bodybuilders. They have to be so spot on with their training, nutrition, and rest to make any kind of gains. Even then, the gains come so slow that natural bodybuilders have to be some of the most patient people on earth. Dieting is also much harder on natural athletes, because in addition to the misery of all the cardio and low carbs, they have to sit and watch a lot of their size and fullness disappear as they get in shape. I was there many times, and it sucked ass. Basically both sides need to have a little more tolerance and respect for the other. We're all bodybuilders, and it's a small enough sport as it is.

Will you ever come out and admit all this, or is this anonymous interview as close as you'll get?

I haven't made any claims about being natural since I wasn't. All the people close to me know. But as far as going on record in a magazine, I don't see what purpose that would serve. The bottom line is that steroids are illegal, and the media has portrayed them in such a way that users are reviled as criminals. I don't see anything positive coming out of a tell-all confession of that sort. I don't want to come off as being proud of using steroids, because I'm not. I'm not really ashamed either, but I think some people would be quick to pass judgement. Who wants that? I don't need all that negativity.

Well, thanks for being as candid as you were.

You're welcome. I hope I was able to get what I learned from my experiences across.

Since then, I have done several more cycles and I don't regret a single one. I know what I am doing, I am a mature, responsible adult, and steroids are a training aid I employ about half the year to reach my physique goals. Now I have 'come out of the closet!'

What Society Thinks About Steroid Users

Steroid users will never be accepted by society, and frankly, I don't even care anymore. The average slob with a potbelly who is too lazy to do any kind of exercise and eats pure shit day after day will dismiss steroid users as lazy cheaters. They will assume anyone in any kind of physical condition must be juicing. After all, there couldn't possibly be any hard work and dedication involved. Ironic, isn't it? Those fools can all kiss my ass. They know only the lies fed to them by the media, and that's all they want to believe. I have had my share of lectures from personal physicians when I confided in them of my history of steroid use. All reacted as I fully expected them to, which was to tell me I was going to die very soon if I didn't stop using these deadly drugs. I challenged each of them to quote me some statistics of all the deaths caused directly from steroid use. They couldn't come up with any, of course. Yet these same doctors have no qualms writing prescriptions for powerful drugs to balance out your moods, keep your penis hard, kill pain, or help you sleep. All of those drugs have inherent dangers and side effects, including death, but they all enjoy a pristine reputation in comparison to steroids. Basically, don't ever expect anyone you know to accept or understand your steroid use, because they won't. They have been programmed for years to believe steroids are deadly, evil, and a pox on society. Don't waste your time trying to convince them otherwise, as these beliefs have been instilled as powerfully as religious doctrine.

Your Training And Nutrition Will Always Be More Important Than The Drugs You Use

This may sound like a reiteration of what has already been discussed so far, but the one point I want to make sure I drive home is that steroids are nothing more than a "supplement" to hard training and diligent eating. I believe the Internet has confused a great deal of the current generation of bodybuilders, particularly the younger guys. While there is a lot of information provided and exchanged about training and nutrition, the hunger for knowledge about steroids and endless discussions about how to use them optimally has become ravenous. If you posted an article about how Mr. Olympia trains, then posted another with which dugs he uses and detailing the whole cycle, I guarantee you the second article would get a hundred times more hits. When I try and downplay the role of steroids in the sum total of a champion physique, I am inevitably met with sarcasm and ridicule from the "message board" generation. They honestly think I am trying to thwart them from achieving their goals by deterring them from the Holy Grail – more and more steroids. The worst thing I see happening is the explosion of online "gurus" counseling others on how to use steroids. These anonymous figures often have screen names like "TestKing315" or "2HugeTrenLover," and will often pass themselves off of 280 pounds and ripped. In fact, many times they are average-looking guys who read enough about steroids to sound like they know what they are talking about. In most cases, I bet the guys asking their advice are built better than their online drug coach. The dangerous thing here is that most of these gurus are taken at face value as experts, and their clients will do as they are told. If the guru outlines a stack that has the bodybuilder shooting two grams of test a week, a gram of deca, 10 iu's of GH a day, and three Anadrols a day, the bodybuilder will do it without question. It's easy to see the danger here. When the bodybuilder doesn't see the gains he or she was expecting, the guru, who knows very little about training and nutrition, will simply tell them to up the dosages. That is always the answer. Or, if the client isn't losing as much bodyfat as they wanted to, the directive will be to take more clenbuterol, more T-3, and more DNP. This is all a recipe for disaster, as the potential for health problems rises with the amount of drugs a person takes. Some of the pro's do in fact take outrageous amounts of drugs, but some of them do not. The scant few who will actually talk about the amounts they use get blasted by fans as liars when the dosages aren't as crazy as they imagined. Lee Priest is a great example. Many bodybuilding fans that are envious of his incredible muscular thickness refuse to believe he is being truthful when he goes on record and details exactly how much he uses, which is a very modest amount even compared to most amateurs. But it is hard for these fans to admit that Lee looks the way he does not because of the drugs he takes. Certainly they do play a supporting role. But it is his gifted genetics and many years of hard training that made Lee Priest's physique so extraordinary and awe-inspiring. Admitting that hurts too much to someone who has obviously not inherited similar genetics and is not willing to put in all those years of workouts and regular meals. But I assure you, steroids have not and will never make a champion out of the average Joe who has normal genetics and who doesn't train and eat at a level superior to 99% of the men and women in any gym.

Synthol – Who Are You Fooling?

Lastly, I want to discuss the substance known as Synthol, which was actually only briefly a trade name of the first commercially available 'site-enhancment oil' that has spread throughout a sport over the past few years. Just as we call all brands of facial tissues Kleenex and all diapers are Pampers, so has Synthol become the universal name for all of these products. Without getting too technical (since I can't anyway), Synthol is nothing more than sterilized MCT oil (hopefully sterilized) and some local painkiller like lidocaine (similar to Novocain). It is sold as a 'posing oil' at anywhere from 100 to 300 dollars for a 50 ml bottle. It is actually used by some bodybuilders to inject into weak muscle groups to give instant size – effectively an oil implant. It is generally used on smaller bodyparts like the biceps, triceps, and calves, though you also see a few that inject into the shoulders or even the chest. Synthol is also regarded by many in the sport as being a blight on bodybuilding, a blatant case of cheating even to those who use all manner of muscle-building and fat-burning drugs.

The whole argument against Synthol is that although steroids definitely assist in building muscle size, you still have to work to make the gains. Nobody ever got a twenty-inch arm by shooting steroids and not bothering to work out. However, there have been more than a few Synthol users who were able to graduate from arms in the very human 16-18-inch range to 20-23-inch guns in a span of weeks or a couple months, with no actual muscle growth taking place, only the accumulation of oil in pockets inside the muscles, and no extra training involved. As you may ascertain from the previous description, the visual effects of Synthol are not always aesthetically pleasing. The end result is often a mutated-looking arm or shoulder, with oddly shaped lumps and bumps. Sometimes the muscle even takes on impossible shapes and angles that God never had in mind when he designed us. Only the most skilled and judicious use of Synthol users are fooling anyone, but they make up a small percentage of the total. Most users get greedy and keep putting more and more oil into the same area as they see the instant size and crave more. They often lose sight of what they are doing and go overboard. Before they realize what they are doing looks really stupid and fake, it's too late. How long does Synthol remain inside a muscle? I have heard everything from a couple months, to a couple years, to forever. I think the correct answer is probably right in the middle. So you get yourself some tumorous looking 21-inch arms between normal-sized shoulders and delts. All of us 'in the know' in bodybuilding laugh our asses off at you. It looks stupid, and in no way naturally-occurring. Synthol is totally obvious, so its users become instant laughingstocks. Of course, there are a couple of the more famous users of site enhancement oil who don't seem to care whether they are scorned or ridiculed, so long as they are famous. For the record, the best-known alleged Synthol user, Gregg Valentino, claims along with his personal physician that his arms contain no Synthol. His arms are supposedly the product of injecting thousands of milliters of steroids into his arms over a course of years. But whatever is responsible, he is widely ridiculed and even hated by many bodybuilders.

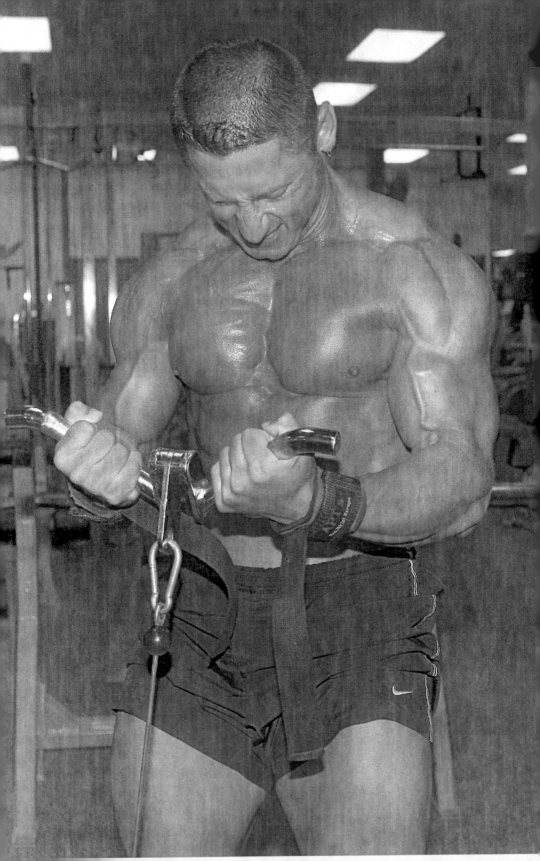

04

HARDCORE TRAINING – GET READY TO WORK, AND TO GROW!

Training is a complex subject, and many books have been written about it. In this chapter, I will summarize my thoughts and offer what I have learned through over two decades of research, observation, and personal experience. I have broken it down into three major areas: how to gain muscular bodyweight, how to sustain motivation and intensity over the long term, and how to avoid overtraining. After that, we address a subject that should always be included in discussions on training – safety and injury.

Gaining Weight

Before we begin, I will clarify what I mean by gaining weight. What we are talking about is muscular bodyweight, not just fat. Anyone can sit on a sofa, eat junk all day and night, and sure enough they will see a large increase in bodyweight. I'm sure that you are not looking to gain this type of weight. You want muscle mass: bigger thicker arms, legs, chest, back, shoulders, a look of power that instantly tells everyone who sees you that you are a big, strong person. As a former short, skinny runt who used to be beat up, stuffed into lockers at school, then thrown into thorny bushes on the way home by bullies, becoming large and muscular was something I dreamed about for years. Once I discovered weight training, I searched relentlessly for any information that could help me gain weight. I started training at age 15 at 90 pounds soaking wet, and by the time I was 22 I was tipping the scales at 230 pounds, without the use of any drugs whatsoever. The muscle didn't exactly pile on right away. Many of the pro's and top amateur bodybuilders I have spoken to were asked if they lifted weights several years before they ever did. I had been training for several years before anyone seemed to notice any extra size. The rate of the gains I made in weight had a direct correlation with the level of knowledge I acquired. In fact, the last forty pounds came in less than two years, and in that time I had been working in Los Angeles in the bodybuilding industry. Since then, I have written extensively and personally coached dozens of men and women on the subject of gaining weight. It's not rocket science, but without the right plan gaining weight can be nearly impossible for a lot of people. No matter how hard it has been up until now for you to gain weight, I can tell you with full confidence that the pounds will start coming as soon as you read this and begin applying the principles I will outline. First, let's examine the whole subject of being a "hardgainer" so you can have a better idea where you truly stand.

What Is A "Hardgainer?"

The term "hardgainer" became popular in the bodybuilding world about ten years ago through the writings of Stuart McRobert, who published a magazine of the same name from the island of Cyprus. It came to symbolize anyone who felt that results from training were much more difficult for them to come by than for the average person. Soon, we had hundreds of thousands of men around the world who had labeled themselves hardgainers. I was one of them, I confess. McRobert eventually changed the term to "genetically average" to more accurately reflect the truth. The reality is that bonafide hardgainers are just as rare as genetic superiors. Just as there aren't many guys who start training and become heavily muscled within a year, there are very few people who can train and eat right without seeing at least average results. But, since a lot of people don't really know what they're doing in regards to training and nutrition, they blame their meager gains on terrible genetics. Another thing that causes many trainers to leap to the conclusion that they are hardgainers is comparing themselves to genetic superiors. Listen, in comparison to freaks like Ronnie Coleman or Flex

Wheeler, we're all hardgainers! Look at the big picture for a minute. Take your gym, for example. How many guys there look like anything like the bodybuilders in the magazines? I'd venture not more than a handful at the majority of gyms, if that. How many guys have been there for a year or more training consistently, yet still look as if they have yet to lift their first weight? I bet there aren't many of those either. 90 % of the people at your gym probably look like they work out, but they are nothing to look twice at. They are genetically average. Not genetically cursed, or hardgainers, just average. If they did more things right in the gym and with their eating and recovery, they would no doubt look a whole lot better. The odds are enormously in favor of you being genetically average as well. You might be closer to the low or high end of average, but chances are you are indeed in the huge portion of the genetic pie chart that qualifies you as average. The lesson here is that just because your results aren't as fast as you would like by no means makes you a hardgainer. Adding muscular bodyweight is not a rapid process, especially when you're doing it naturally, which is the safest and most lasting way to do it. If it was so quick and easy, we would have a lot more big people walking around. Because it takes such a long time to build an above-average amount of muscle, most people give up in frustration rather quickly. If they knew the right things to do, they would make gains at the fastest rate possible. As I say, the more you know, the more you grow.

Realistic Expectations

How much weight can you expect to gain? A few factors come into play here. One is, how much weight have you already gained? If you started at 150 and are only 160 a year later, it's safe to say you have plenty of room to grow, anywhere from 20 to 50 more pounds eventually. If you started at 150 and you're 200 pounds five years later, you probably don't have fifty more pounds left in your natural genetic potential. All these numbers are fairly irrelevant, as no one can accurately predict how much muscle mass you are ultimately capable of building. One thing that is certain is that if you haven't gained much muscle at all yet, you have a lot of growth potential still untapped.

The Magic Trio

To gain weight, you must carefully control three areas: training, nutrition (which includes supplementation), and rest. Listen carefully to this next sentence. *All three of these areas must be maximized at all times, or your results will be less than optimal.* Even if your training is perfect and you eat the right foods at the right times, you will not synthesize much new muscle tissue if you stay out all night and miss sleep, or train every day. If you eat right and get plenty of rest but your training isn't sufficiently intense to stimulate gains, again little will happen. And even if you train right and get plenty of rest, yet neglect to fuel your body with the proper nutrients at regular intervals, once more your gains will be less than thrilling. Think of these three areas as sides to a pyramid. If any one side is weak, the whole structure crumbles. You must decide right now that you will pay equal attention to all three, because they are all essential components to reaching your goal. Never let yourself think that extra attention to one or two sides of the triangle will make up for slacking off in the third. It won't. With that key point made, let's get into the nuts and bolts of gaining weight, focusing on one area at a time.

Training To Gain Weight

Luckily, there is no mystery as to how to train to gain as much muscle mass as possible. Millions before us have done all the experimenting over many decades, and the proven free weight basics are primarily what will pack on the beef. This is not to say that certain machines do not have a place in your training, even when pure size is your number one priority. The trick is in knowing when free weights will do the job best and when a machine can do it as well or better. In some cases, a pre-existing injury will make certain free weight movements difficult to perform with sufficient weight. If, for instance, you have a herniated disk in your lower back, heavy squats or deadlifts are definitely out of the question. Though squats are excellent for building the entire lower body and stimulating the metabolism, you can still get very good results from other exercises. Let's run down the best free weight exercises for each bodypart before we proceed.

Back	• Deadlift • Barbell row • Chin-up • One-arm row • Barbell or dumbbell shrugs
Legs	• Squats • Stiff-leg deadlift
Chest	• Barbell or dumbbell flat bench press • Barbell or dumbbell incline bench press • Barbell or dumbbell decline bench press • Weighted dips, leaning forward • Dumbbell flyes, flat, incline, or decline
Shoulders	• Seated press, barbell or dumbbells • Side raise • Barbell upright row
Biceps	• Barbell curl • Alternate dumbbell curl • Reverse barbell curl • Hammer-grip dumbbell curl
Triceps	• Weighted dips, torso upright • Close-grip bench press • Lying barbell extension, flat or decline bench • Seated single dumbbell extension

Equal Attention To All

It shouldn't have to be said, but you must train all your major muscle groups, especially the legs, back, and chest, if you want to make any meaningful improvements in total body muscle mass and weight. Too many trainers focus most of their attention on "show muscles" like the chest and arms, not realizing that this is a pathetically ineffective way to gain weight. I have seen this a thousand times. Two young guys with near-equal genetics start training at the same time. One trains only his chest and arms, and gets some size in both. However, he only gains a few pounds of weight. The other guy trains hard on squats, deadlifts, rows, bench presses, shoulder presses, chin-ups, and weighted dips, making an effort to use more and more weight whenever he can. This guy gets big all over, looking like one strong dude, and gains so much muscular weight that old friends barely recognize him, and none of his old clothes fit anymore. And his chest and arms are at least as good as the first guy or better, except he also has powerful lats, shoulders, and legs to match. Putting most of your effort into training the large muscle groups is the only way you will ever see large increases in total body mass. They are where the potential for significant gains truly resides. If you either skip or just do a couple half-ass sets for any of them, understand that you are short-changing yourself from the gains you could be making.

How Many Reps?

Many studies have confirmed that the best rep range to stimulate muscle growth is 8-12 for the upper body, and 12-20 for the lower body, which has more slow-twitch muscle fibers. Powerlifters have also shown that using lower reps over many sets, such as ten sets of 3-5 reps in the bench press, will also stimulate growth. The reason I will not go into this style of training is that for most people, three to five reps is too dangerous to do on a regular basis. The resistance is too heavy to handle safely and in correct form. Additionally, I believe everyone has to develop that mind-muscle connection, that deep feeling and control of your muscular contractions, to reach their ultimate potential. It's much harder, if not impossible, for most people to develop that feeling and connection while using very heavy weights.

Training To Failure – The Only Assurance Of Proper Intensity

Pushing your body to its limits and beyond is the only way you will force it to grow new muscle tissue. We do this by taking a set to the point where no further reps are possible, despite our maximum effort. So when I say to do 8-12 reps on the barbell bench press, for example, the weight must be heavy enough so that you reach failure in that range. If you can only do five or six, take a bit of weight off. If you get more than twelve, you need to add a bit more weight. The only sets that should not be taken to failure are warm-ups. Do not waste a lot of time and energy on warm-ups. Always precede any weight training session with five to seven moderate-pace minutes on any piece of cardio equipment to raise your body's core temperature, then start your warmups. Say your best bench press for eight reps is with 225 pounds (two 45-pound plates). Your first warm-up should be with the bar for ten very easy, slow reps to get accustomed to the movement pattern. Your second set should be with 135 (one plate a side) for no more than eight reps. Finally, load up 185 for just four reps. Now you're ready to start your work sets, with plenty of blood in the chest and shoulders, yet you haven't depleted any strength.

Pyramid Up Or Down?

Should you start with your heaviest weight and work down, or instead add weight for each of your sets as they go on? Both ways have their pros and cons. Starting with your heaviest weight allows you to use the greatest amount of resistance when your strength and energy levels are highest. Someone who works up to 200 pounds for eight reps over three or four sets probably could use 220 or more for eight reps if they went to it right after warming up. A series of bench press sets like this would look something like this:

Set 1:   225 x 8
Set 2:   215 x 8
Set 3:   205 x 8

Greater resistance does equate to more mass gains. Personally, I believe this method is best for those with several years of lifting experience under their belts already. The other option is to add weight and drop reps as the sets go on. A bench press session in that format for the same person could look like this:

Set 1: 175 x 12
Set 2: 190 x 9
Set 3: 205 x 8

Pyramiding up is safer and gives you more time to acclimate yourself to the heavier weights, but it does not allow you to use as much resistance as starting heavy and pyramiding down. Both methods will produce results. It's simply a matter of personal preference and what you feel comfortable with. Many people can't just jump into a heavy weight, while others feel like they're wasting time and holding back if they take several sets to get to their heaviest weight on an exercise. Try it both ways if you haven't already, and one will just feel more right for you.

Good Form – Make Sure The Muscles Are Under Tension

All this talk about using heavy weights has to be followed up with a discussion of good form. You must use the heaviest weights you can handle, but only if you can handle them in good form. Cheating and heaving weights up is bad for two critical reasons. One, it's a sure-fire way to get injured. You may never have had a training injury, so you might not realize just how devastating they can be. A serious injury to the lower back, rotator cuffs of the shoulder, a muscle tear, or even inflamed tendons in the elbows or knees can limit or in some cases even stop your training for many months. That's time you could be getting bigger, but if you're injured you'll just be shrinking back down to normal size. Second, bad form actually prevents the muscle you're trying to work from getting any meaningful stimulation. Let's use barbell curls as an example. We have all seen guys who use far too much weight on this exercise. You might even have done this yourself, or still do it. The barbell curl is supposed to isolate the biceps, but when you heave it up with a hip thrust and bend backwards to get it up, it's more front delts and lower back moving the weight. A cheat curl is more similar to an Olympic lift like a snatch than it is a bodybuilding exercise. In cheating style, the biceps are only under tension for a split second somewhere in the middle of the movement. Now think of a strict barbell curl. The torso is upright, the elbows are pinned to the sides. All that moves is the upper arms as they slowly bring the weight up solely by contracting the biceps. The cheat curler may have been able to fling up 150 pounds, but his biceps probably aren't anything special. Show me someone who can curl 150 pounds in strict style, and his biceps are going to look like two softballs are stuffed into his upper arms. Is a little cheating okay? There is indeed a time and a place for cheating. When no more strict reps are possible, it's fine to extend the set with a cheat rep or two. Certain exercises, like curls, laterals for the shoulders, and cable pushdowns are well suited for cheat reps. Others, like squats, overhead presses, or deadlifts, could be very dangerous to use loose form on. As a general rule, exercises that employ heavier loads are not suited for cheat reps.

Tension on the muscle is what you must always strive to maximize. The old Nautilus guideline of two seconds up, four seconds down was excellent at minimizing momentum and forcing good form. I would say a fine alternative that will let you use more weight yet still keeps the form tight is two seconds up, a half-second to squeeze the muscle at the contraction point (what Joe Weider calls the Peak Contraction Principle), and two seconds to lower the weight. You might have to count inside your head for a little while to get the feel for this rep tempo, but soon it will come naturally as you get used to it. The squeeze is very important, as it makes the major difference between training a muscle and just lifting a weight from point A to point B. It also makes a huge difference in how well you stimulate the muscle to grow. A lot of clients I worked with over the years found it helpful to say the word "squeeze" as they lifted the weight, and "stretch" as they lowered it. Basically, this is all we really do with weights – shorten and lengthen a muscle or group of muscles. A final note on squeezing; some exercises are not compatible with such an emphasis on contractions. Squats and deadlifts are probably the only two movements during which attempting to contract your muscles at the end of the rep would actually detract from your performance, as both exercises need a tremendous amount of skill and concentration to properly execute.

Isolation Movements?

To gain serious mass, the emphasis has to be on basic movements that allow you to work the big muscle groups with a lot of weight. This means that isolation, or so-called "shaping" movements don't have a legitimate place in this phase of your training. You only have a very limited amount of "gas" any time you train, so don't waste your energy on ten sets on the pec dec or leg extensions. Those movements all have their place later on, but we must keep them to a bare minimum during your major gaining period. Don't worry that your arms or calves are going to shrink. When you hit the big bodyparts, the smaller ones are also very much involved. There's no way to row a 300-pound barbell without working your biceps hard, or bench press 350 pounds without plenty of work for the triceps. In the routines I will now outline, I have included only the exercises for the smaller bodyparts that belong. Do *not* add any more exercises or sets, or you threaten to compromise the effectiveness of this routine. If you are unsure of how to do any of these exercises, either hire an experienced personal trainer to show you, or follow the instructions in my course pertaining to that bodypart.

Routine A – Three Days a Week

Monday	Flat barbell or dumbbell bench press	4 x 8-12
	Squats	4 x 12-20
	Barbell rows	4 x 8-12
	Barbell curls	3 x 8-12
Wednesday	Chin-ups	4 x 8-12 (add weight if needed)
	Overhead barbell or dumbbell press	4 x 8-12
	Stiff-leg deadlifts	4 x 8-12
	(Note: hamstrings have recently been found to react better to rep ranges traditionally suited to the upper body, while quadriceps still need higher reps)	
	Leg curls	4 x 12-20
Friday	Deadlifts	4 x 8-12
	Weighted dips	4 x 8-12
	Lying triceps extensions	3 x 8-12
	Standing calf raise	3 x 12-20
	Crunches	3 x 12-20 (hold weight if needed)

Routine B – Variation on Three Days a Week

Day One	Incline barbell or dumbbell bench press	4 x 8-12
	Weighted dips	4 x 8-12
	Overhead press	4 x 8-12
	Barbell or alternate dumbbell curl	4 x 8-12
Day Two	Squats	4 x 12-20
	Stiff-leg deadlifts	4 x 8-12
	Leg curls	4 x 8-12
	Standing calf raise	4 x 12-20
Rest		
Day Three	Deadlifts	4 x 8-12
	Chin-ups	4 x 8-12
	Barbell or dumbbell row	4 x 8-12
	Barbell or dumbbell shrugs	4 x 8-12
Rest one day, begin again with day one		

Routine C – Push, Pull, Legs

Day One – Pushing Muscles	Flat bench press	4 x 8-12
	Overhead press	4 x 8-12
	Seated single dumbbell extension	4 x 8-12
	Weighted dips	4 x 8-12
Rest one day		
Day Two – Pulling Muscles	Deadlifts	4 x 8-12
	Chin-ups	4 x 8-12
	Barbell rows	4 x 8-12
	Upright rows	3 x 8-12
	Shrugs	3 x 8-12
	Barbell or preacher curl	3 x 8-12
Rest one day		
Day Three – Legs	Squats	5 x 12-20
	Leg curls	5 x 8-12
	Stiff-leg deadlifts	5 x 8-12
	Standing calf raise	4 x 12-20
Rest one day, repeat cycle		

Substitutions?

The only case where it is permissible to substitute exercises is if a pre-existing injury would make it too dangerous to execute. For instance, if you can't safely perform squats, leg presses will do. If you can't deadlift with an Olympic bar, try using a Gerard trap bar or dumbbells. Definitely do not substitute machine movements simply because they are easier to perform. It is the difficulty of the free weight staples that forces your body to work so hard and grow. You can design your own routines if you keep the focus on the mass-builders and allow time for individual bodyparts to recover. For instance, you would not want to deadlift and squat on the same day, or even on two consecutive days. Both exercises place a great deal of stress on the lower back. If you are unsure about which exercises might overlap in terms of muscle groups, I advise you to follow one of the above three routines exactly as it is outlined. They might seem very basic, but it's hard work on the basics that delivers the best results. Everyone I have ever put on one of these type of routines has grown bigger and stronger at a much faster rate than when they followed a more traditional split routine, training one bodypart a day with mostly isolation exercises. When you have built a solid base of muscle mass, then you can start worrying about shaping and refining it.

A Note On Cardio

During your period of weight gain, avoid all cardiovascular activity. More on that when we discuss resting to gain weight.

Resting To Gain Weight

Now we come to the final side of the triangle, rest and recovery. Overtraining should not be a problem as long as you stick fairly close to one of the training routines outlined earlier. These are designed to give not only the individual muscle groups enough time to rebuild, but your nervous system as well. The most important component of your recovery is getting enough sleep. Eight hours is the bare minimum per night. I realize that with work, school, and family responsibilities in many of your lives, this might even be pushing reality. Do your best to get as much sleep as you can. If you are able to get nine or ten hours a night, do it. If you can take a nap during the day, do that as well. If your weeknights are tough to manage more than six or seven hours, try to make up for it on the weekends. Whatever you do, don't stay out all hours of the night partying when you could be at home resting and growing from your last workout. Most of the regenerative processes of our bodies, including muscle repair and growth, occur during sleep. Missing out on sleep will severely hamper your gains. I can't make it any clearer than that. Flex Wheeler made his best progress in his last two years as an amateur (growing from a light-heavyweight to a heavyweight), and not coincidentally he was sleeping up to sixteen hours a day for most of that time.

Minimizing Extra Activities

The late Peary Rader, who started *Ironman* magazine over 65 years ago, had a phrase that I think perfectly sums up how someone trying to gain muscle should manage their energy. I'm paraphrasing, but the gist of it is, "Never run when you can walk, never walk when you can stand, never stand when you can sit, and never sit when you can lie down." Essentially he was saying to conserve as much energy as possible so that there would be nothing to compete with the energy reserves needed to train and recover from training. Especially if gaining weight has been a huge challenge for you, it is imperative that you limit any extra physical activities to a bare minimum. Playing sports, rollerblading, biking, even hours of dancing at a club will all take away from your energy reserves. I am basically telling you to be a lazy slug except when you're training with weights. This won't be as easy if you work a physical job such as construction, but do the best you can. Whenever you see a chance to lay down or even better, to catch a little nap, don't hesitate. Just as you want to take in a bit more calories than you really need, you should strive to get more sleep than you need also. This program is going to place tremendous metabolic demands on your body. The more rest you can get, the better your body will be able to deal with the demands and meet the challenge by growing bigger and stronger.

Putting It All Together

The triangle is complete. Now you know everything you need to about how to train, eat, and rest to gain muscular bodyweight. The ball is in your court. If you follow the instructions to the T, you can expect to start making some excellent gains within just two or three weeks. If you slack in any one of the three areas, your gains will not be as good as they could be. If you have that burning desire to be a bigger, stronger you, bursting with powerful muscle mass, then it's time to get to work. Dedicate yourself to sticking to this program 100 %, and very soon the new you will be under construction. Remember, expect more from yourself, don't make any excuses, and go for it! See you in the land of big men soon.

Motivation and Intensity

I can sum up the core of generating motivation and intensity by asking one question: how bad do you want it? Desire is the foundation of all you will do in weight training or bodybuilding. How well you will be able to sustain the motivation to train with high intensity over the months and years is directly proportional to how badly you want to change your physique. I would even go so far as to say that you should feel like you absolutely *must* improve your body or else your life will not be complete. While others can debate how healthy a mindset this is, there is no question that the most highly motivated individuals do not sit around and say things like, "well, it would be nice to be a little bigger or stronger, but it's no big deal if I don't." This is how most people you see in the gym are. They want to improve, but not so much that they're willing to work hard for it. You could compare them to most Americans who would like to be wealthy, but don't want to go out of their way by working hard and taking risks to do so. When desire and determination are strong enough, there is virtually nothing that can stop someone from making their dreams a reality. We are all familiar with stories of those who started out dirt-poor, yet through perseverance, hard work, and sacrifice, amassed great wealth. These people wanted to succeed so much that they refused to give up, no matter how bleak things may have looked at times or how many obstacles might have blocked their path. Think about that, because it isn't so different from making changes with your body.

90 % of the "success stories" that result from weight training have nothing to do with contests or titles. By far, most of the successes are people who started out underweight or overweight, and made sincere efforts to craft their bodies into what they knew they were capable of. Bill Phillips has made this process famous by packaging and marketing it into an ongoing "Body For Life" transformation contest. Every month in *Muscle Media* magazine, you used to read stories about people who were fed up with their present physical condition, and decided to do something about it right away. As Anthony Robbins might say, they knew a change was needed, and they recognized that they were the only ones who could make it happen.

Why Do You Want To Change?

I will assume that you want to change, or else you wouldn't have come this far. Now you have to get very specific. What changes, exactly, do you want to make, and why? Right now, get a piece of paper and make two columns. In one column, put your goals. In the second, list the reasons you want to achieve those goals. Here's an example of what that might look like.

Goals	Reasons to Achieve
Lose four inches from my waistline	Feel more confident, less self-conscious about taking shirt off
	Fit into nicer clothes
	Have a better V-taper
Gain an inch on my arms	Feel more confident in short sleeves
	Feel more powerful, virile
	Impress that girl at the gym I like

Obviously, you will have your own goals. But notice some things about the two hypothetical columns. The goals were very specific, and that's important. Rather than say that you want to lose some fat or gain some muscle, you quantify exactly how much and from where. The more detailed and specific you make your goals, the better your odds of achieving them. This is because you have a distinct destination. Once you have that destination, your brain starts searching for ways to get there. It's like taking a vacation. If you have no idea where you want to go or only a vague idea, you'll probably end up staying home and watching TV on your vacation. But if you know you want to go to a specific place like Jamaica, you'll start looking into airline tickets and hotel reservations. With your body, having goals to measure is critical. You will always have a more clear direction when you say, "I want to gain five pounds of muscle by December 1st," than if you say "I'd like to put some muscle on this fall." Because how much is some? An ounce? A pound? Ten pounds? You see what I mean. Use very specific terms when outlining your goals. The reasons you want to achieve your goals must also be detailed, as well as honest. Don't worry that reasons such as wanting to impress your old classmates at a high school reunion or trying to catch the eye of an aerobics instructor at the gym are selfish or juvenile. If these are the things that excite and inspire you, never fear that your motivations aren't good enough. This list is for your eyes only. If you are going to put a great deal of hard work and time into any endeavor, you have to believe that the reward is going to make it all worth it. Think of the rewards you would really love to receive. What do you feel a more muscular body would do for you, inside and out? These are the things that are going to keep you going.

Here's an example of a set of goals and rewards that has been working wonders for decades. Many young men in their teens suffer from low self-esteem and a feeling of not being accepted by the group (their peers). Thus, usually after seeing a muscular man in real life or in some form of media, they get the idea in their heads that if they too could become big and strong, everything in their lives would be better. They believe that being muscular would earn them the respect and admiration of their male peers, as well as make them far more desirable to the opposite sex. Since these are the two driving goals of most adolescent males, motivation is not usually a problem when they decide to start weight training. They will train with any equipment available, at any hours they can, and do their best to lift more and more weight all the time. Teenage men are some of the most enthusiastic trainers you will ever hope to find, simply because they know what they want, they want it very badly, and they want it *now*. You will never hear a teenager say, "well, I want to start lifting, but I think I'll wait until after the holidays this year." Not on your life. A teenager will beg, borrow, or steal to somehow get to some equipment or a gym as soon as possible. There is a valuable lesson to be learned from what drives them. If you can tap into the emotions deep down inside that make you want to change, your motivation will have that much more power. Really, the bottom line is that we all want to feel better about ourselves. You need to be honest with yourself and determine what you really want out of weight training or bodybuilding. Your own goals may be as simple as putting on twenty pounds or to win a local contest, but be very clear on what your goals are and why you want to achieve them.

Principles Of Motivation

Now that you know what you want and why you want it, it's time to give you some specific strategies on how to foster that motivation. Let's face it, negativity is a very easy state to fall into, and doing nothing is always much easier than doing something. Here are some ways to make sure you are always moving toward your goals.

Set Deadlines To Create A Sense Of Urgency

Contests, whether they be actual competitions on stage or supplement company "before and after" transformations, are excellent because they force a limited time frame within which to reach your peak condition. Nearly all of us are procrastinators by nature. If we don't have to do something immediately, particularly something that entails significant effort, we will put it off as long as possible. With no special time or date to worry about, people do things like miss workouts, have half-ass workouts, miss meals, or neglect to eat the right foods at the right times. After all, what's the big deal, right? They can always go to the gym and have a better workout some other day, or start eating more protein and less junk next week. This is how most people operate, and it's why you see them looking exactly the same, if not worse, year after year in the gym. What if you suddenly apply a deadline of say, ten weeks to reach top condition? Immediately, everything takes on a sense of **urgency**. Urgency is your friend, because it stirs you to action. If you wake up and have to decide whether to go to the gym or blow it off, that sense of urgency tells you that you don't have time to blow off any training. Every day counts. Once you get to the gym, that same sense of urgency will drive you to train your hardest, pushing for more weight, more reps, more intense cardio. Instead of catching some cruddy bite to eat at Wendy's, you'll be eating chicken breasts, potatoes, vegetables, and other forms of proper fuel. In your mind at all times will be a ticking clock, counting down the time you have left to achieve your goal. It's this type of pressure that brings out the best in all of us.

The deadline doesn't have to entail a contest. It could be something as simple as a vacation to the Bahamas, or even looking good for the start of the beach season. Women do this all the time, going on crash diets and embarking on workout regimens so that they can be thin for weddings, class reunions, vacations, and swimsuit seasons. High school football players in certain positions often need to gain a certain amount of bodyweight over the summer vacation to be considered for starting positions on the varsity squad that fall. Many recreational bodybuilders even make appointments with a professional photographer to take studio posing shots on a certain day, paying in advance. These types of deadlines are usually best, because you can't change them. Since you can't change the date, you have to do whatever it takes to change yourself in the allotted time period. Also, shorter time frames work best. I would any more than three months or so is going to make it harder to maintain your focus and motivation. Longer time periods also remove a great deal of the sense of urgency, since you can always assume there will still be time to 'get on the ball' even if you start slacking off. That may work in college courses where you can "cram" right before finals, but the body doesn't work like that. With periods of four, six, or ten weeks, there's no time for slacking off whatsoever.

Establish A Rivalry

Another great way of fueling your motivation is to have a rivalry with someone. Since most of you won't be going neck-and-neck with Ronnie Coleman, a better choice would be to either make a bet with a friend regarding who can get better results in a given time frame, or start training with someone who you already have some sort of rivalry with. This works great for men because we are ego and pride-driven creatures. When I trained with *Ironman* cover model Steve Cuevas back in the mid 90's, we both had some of the most intense training sessions of our lives. We were both two of Southern California's best natural bodybuilders at the time, and every day in the gym it was a battle to see who could out-do the other. We challenged ourselves to lift more weight, get more reps, and go further past the pain zone than the other guy, and we both improved quite a bit in just a couple months. The balance was always shifting, since we both had advantages over the other in certain areas. I also used to enjoy training with guys on steroids, though I wasn't. I was determined to out-train them regardless of any chemical advantage, and that forced me to dig down deep and pull out every last bit of energy and power that I had. I looked forward to every single workout as another chance to prove myself superior. Rivalries are perfect motivating tools because they actually give you someone to beat other than yourself. It's easy to give up and not care about out-doing your own best efforts, but our pride and ego make it much more difficult to let someone else show us up. Don't be concerned that this is childish or immature. The top CEO's of the Fortune 500 companies play this same scenario out every day on golf courses and tennis courts. Use it in the gym to keep you motivated, focused, and intense.

Photos

We are all visual creatures (especially us men), and photographs of ourselves are especially good at stimulating our emotions. If you used to be in much better shape, tack up the photos of that time somewhere you'll see them constantly, like your refrigerator or office. You could also put up pictures of someone who inspires you, or whose physique you would like yours to resemble. Another way to use pictures is as a visual progress report. Every month on the same day, take pictures in the same lighting conditions and place, if possible. This will either affirm your constant progress, or alert you to a lack of progress that needs to be addressed. When I was in college and really getting obsessed with wanting to be a bodybuilder, my wall was literally papered with full-page cut-outs from the bodybuilding magazines. Every night before I went to sleep I would stare at the collage of bodies of men like Lee Labrada, Rich Gaspari, Lee Haney, Shawn Ray, Mike Mentzer, and Shawn Ray, burning that 'look' into my brain, and programming it to want to look like them.

Visualization

Another tool that can sustain your motivation is to visualize your end result. It's best to do this in a dark and quiet place. Most people do it before they fall asleep, when the mind is especially receptive to this type of exercise. Picture exactly how you want to look. Imagine yourself in the gym, lifting more weight than you now can even dream of. Try to conceive every little detail, using as many senses as possible. Think about not only what you see, but what you hear, smell, feel, etc. This will give you a very lifelike image to save in your memory banks. It will also stimulate your mind to incorporate these images into your dreams, where they will further fuel your motivation and goals. You've heard that anything you can conceive and believe, you can achieve. It's true. The more you reinforce this ideal image of yourself into your conscious and subconscious mind, the easier you will find it to do the things necessary to progress toward this image. It will seem less of a dream after a time and more of a foregone conclusion, needing only you to take the steps to reach it.

Visualization is also a way to make your workouts better. The night before, mentally rehearse the entire training session in your head, noting what you will wear, how strong and confident you will feel, even exactly how many sets and reps you will get with how much weight. Picture yourself grinding out those last nearly impossible reps, getting pumped and feeling on top of the world. At the very least, your workout the next day will be much more focused, since you already planned the whole thing out in your mind beforehand.

Hire A Trainer

If you feel you simply can't bring yourself to stay motivated all the time, hire a personal trainer to give you the occasional shared boost of energy and inspiration. I happen to believe that competitive bodybuilders are best for this assignment, since they train harder than nearly anyone else you will hope to find. They know how to make a training session high-energy, positive, and productive. They are also far less likely to 'baby' a client than most trainers. And of course, their physique should serve as ample motivation for you to train harder.

Belief

The final aspect of motivation to understand and apply is that of belief. To remain highly motivated, you must believe that all your efforts are going to pay off in the long run. This can be tough, because results from weight training are never as fast as we would wish, and sometimes painfully slow. We're so used to seeing dramatic "before and after" pictures in supplement ads that we feel like failures if we can't add thirty pounds of muscle and lose twenty pounds of fat in a month. What most people don't know is that these are almost always people who were already in great shape, and stopped training for a time specifically so that they could go about this wonderful transformation, usually with the goal of winning one of the prizes these contests offer. Steroids are also commonly used to speed up the results. Always keep in mind that you are on a journey, and any journey is made up of small, individual steps. Each step does get you closer to your destination. Every good workout, every good meal, every good night of sleep inches you closer and closer to where you want to be. Because the journey is so long and relatively slow, you will often be tempted to start thinking you will never get there. Banish these negative thoughts. Also be conscious that you will encounter people who want to see you fail because they either never made the effort or gave up themselves. They may try to discourage you, either obviously or through very subtle comments.

Because I was a short and skinny teenager in my early years of training, I had dozens of people tell me I was on a futile quest if I ever thought I was going to be a big, strong man. Since I wanted to be big and strong so much, I simply blocked out these naysayers and kept working toward my goal. Don't let anybody wear you down or make you start doubting yourself. You know where you're headed, you know how to get there, and you know that you will in fact succeed as long as you never quit.

Intensity

What is intensity?

People have different ideas about what intensity means as it applies to weight training and bodybuilding, but here's my definition. Intensity is the degree of effort which you exert. If someone is using a weight that isn't challenging, and their last rep isn't much more difficult than their first rep, their intensity is low. If another person uses a weight that is heavy, and pushes or pulls until they can no longer budge the weight despite their maximum effort, their intensity is high. The chief aim is to train the muscle to momentary muscular failure, the point at which it no longer has the strength to contract. This is the only way to assure progress. Let's use two twins as a model of low and high intensity. Twin A picks up a 50-pound barbell and begins to curl. After 8 reps, the weight starts to feel heavy, and he racks it before he experiences any real discomfort. Twin B picks up a 75-pound barbell and begins to curl. It is heavy right from the start. By the sixth rep, his biceps are starting to burn with lactic acid accumulation and the bar is going up in slow-motion. He grits his teeth, determined to keep going. Somehow he manages a seventh rep, though by now everything in him is telling him enough is enough. But he wants his biceps to grow, and to do that he knows he must force them to go beyond their present capabilities. Closing his eyes and blocking out the pain, he puts every last ounce of effort into that eight rep. It takes a long time to get it up, and he's shaking, but he gets it. Immediately he tries for a ninth rep. The bar gets about an inch up from his waist, and won't move.

He's trying his best to move it, the veins on his biceps popping out like snakes, and his face is beet red. The bar won't move. Twin B racks it, having finished a truly intense set of curls. He knows he did as many reps as he possibly could have – a true high-intensity set.

A large part of training with intensity is using enough weight. Can you train intensely with light weight? The answer is a qualified yes. Doing 100 reps of curls with a 40-pound bar will be very painful and difficult to complete, but the weight is not heavy enough to cause growth. It would be far more 'intense,' from the standpoint of getting bigger and stronger, to take an 80-pound bar and do ten reps to failure. The rep ranges that work for most trainers to become more muscularly massive are 8-12 for the upper body, and 12-20 for the lower. This is a very general rule that has exceptions, but for the most part you can use it as an easy guideline in selecting your weights. To achieve maximum intensity, you must use weights that allow you to fail within these ranges. There are many other intensity techniques that allow you to go further into the pain zone and force the muscles to work harder than otherwise possible. Be aware though, that overuse of these techniques over time can quickly lead to overtraining. Use them sparingly and listen to your body. See the course on avoiding overtraining for more on this subject.

Pre-exhaust

Pre-exhaust is performing an isolation movement for a bodypart, followed immediately by a compound movement that allows other muscles or muscle groups to assist, thus driving the original part into a deeper state of fatigue than otherwise possible. Here are a few examples:

Side lateral raises/overhead presses
Pec dec/bench press
Lat pullover/chin or row
Shrug/upright row
Leg extensions/leg press or squat
Leg curl/stiff-leg deadlift

Some people get upset because they can't use as much weight as usual in the compound movement this way. However, the extra pain and pump should help them understand that they are actually getting more of a benefit. A slightly less effective way to employ pre-exhaust is to do all your sets of the isolation movement before moving on to the compound exercise. You'll still get some of the effect, but not to the degree you would going right from one to the other.

Drop Sets

Drop sets or strip sets are a way of extending the set past its usual boundaries. Say you are leg pressing 500 pounds, and you fail on the fifteenth rep. This doesn't mean that you can't lift anything, only that you are temporarily unable to push 500 pounds. If you took 100 pounds off and kept going, you would probably be able to get at least ten more reps. To get the most out of drop sets, make sure you hit failure before reducing the weight. Otherwise, you're not achieving the highest level of intensity. Also, try to minimize the time it takes to reduce the weight. Machines with weight stacks are obviously the easiest way, though with barbells a training partner can quickly strip off plates. With dumbbells, simply have all the 'bells you'll use in close proximity. How many drops you do is up to you, though with little or no rest, anything beyond three drops will be limited by lactid acid build-up.

Rest-Pause

With credit to the late Mike Mentzer, rest-pause can be a terrific way to up the intensity. How it works is that you finish your set, rest just a few seconds, then pick up the weight again and grind out a couple more reps. This can be repeated as many times as you can still get a rep. It's one way to take a weight you can only get two or three reps with, and instead make eight or ten reps. I have been using this successfully as an integral part of DC Training since June of 2006.

Static Contraction

Static contraction is holding the weight in the contracted position for an extended time as you flex as hard as possible, usually for ten to thirty seconds. If you were doing leg extensions, you would hold your legs in the lockout position and flex your quads with maximum force. The pump and resulting next-day soreness from this are significant.

Supersets

Supersets are going from any one exercise to another with no break in between. Most often the two exercises are for the same bodypart. Pre-exhaust sets would fit into this category, but you could also do two isolation moves for the same bodypart, two compound moves, or two exercises for different bodyparts. Many trainers like to train both biceps and triceps together, supersetting a biceps exercise with one for the triceps. This allows the other muscle group to recover between sets, as well as allowing both muscles to stretch while the other is contracting. Chest and back is another popular superset combination that fits this description.

Giant Sets

Giant sets are three or more exercises performed consecutively with no rest, almost always for the same bodypart. These are brutal and take a lot out of even the most highly conditioned athletes, so use them only occasionally. A superset for the quads might consist of squats, leg extensions, and leg presses. Don't even try these unless you have a good cardiovascular base, or else you'll be gasping for air before you even get to the third exercise.

Forced Reps

Forced reps can be either one of the best training tools in your repertoire, or the worst. A lot of people think they're doing forced reps, but in reality they are relying on a spotter to lift part of the weight for them at all times. You see this most often on the bench press, when trainers can't even get one rep without their partner helping. A true forced rep follows at least a few reps that have been performed entirely on your own, and then the spotter just helps enough to keep the weight moving for a couple more. If you get assistance from the very beginning, it's not a forced rep – it's tag-team lifting. Don't use forced reps all the time. Try using them only on the last set of each exercise.

Cheat Reps

Cheat reps are essentially forced reps by yourself. Since you don't have a partner, you use a little body English to get a couple more reps. Some exercises you never want to do this on, such as squats and deadlifts. The loads are too great, and the risk of injury too high to deviate from proper form for even a rep or two. Other exercises are much more suited to cheat reps. For barbell curls, a little hip thrust and leaning back will allow you to eke out a couple more reps. When chinning, a little kick of the legs can do the same. Like forced reps, be sure that cheat reps are only used after you have already done several strict reps. Otherwise, you won't be training the muscle itself very efficiently.

Extended Sets

Extended sets are a form of superset in which you use the exact same piece of equipment and weight. Usually, you start off with the exercise that's harder to do with that amount of weight. For example, you could do reverse curls with an EZ bar. When you fail with the reverse curls, flip your hands over and proceed to do regular EZ bar curls. Here are some other good combos:
Front squats/back squats
Front raise with barbell/upright row
Reverse-grip cable pushdown/standard cable pushdown
Dumbbell flyes/dumbbell presses

Negative-Accentuated Training

We can all lower far more weight than we are able to lift. Negative-accentuated sets take advantage of this. Negative-only training is also very valuable, but very difficult to do without two strong spotters. You can do negative-accentuated training by yourself. Machines with fixed movement arms are the easiest way. Let's say you're on the leg extension. You raise the weight with both legs, but lower it using only one. When that leg can no longer control the weight from falling, switch to the other leg. It's very tough on the muscles, so make sure they get plenty of rest after this – a week before training them again is about right.

1 1/4's (One And A Quarters)

1 ¼'s are another way to emphasize the contraction. Using the leg extension as an example again, you would do the rep, then only lower it a quarter of the way back down before squeezing up again. That's one rep.

Superslow

Superslow training, which has been patented by a man named Ken Hutchins, involves slowing the rep down to eliminate any momentum or cheating. Most people get the best results taking ten seconds to perform the positive or lifting segment, and five seconds to lower it. It's a way of boosting the intensity (just try dips or chin-ups this way!) but it's also very valuable for times when injury prevents you from using as much weight as normal. Superslow will make 100 pounds feel as heavy as 500.

Stimulants

Most of the products advertised as "fat-burners" are actually more effective, I feel, at stimulating the central nervous system and allowing you to train harder and longer. I take them year-round, whether I'm trying to gain weight or get lean. There are a lot of good products on the market at any time. All can help you become more alert, raise your body temperature and heart rate, and generally put yourself in a condition more agreeable to blasting heavy weights with no fear. If you don't want to use them, a strong cup or two of coffee will deliver a similar effect. There are some things you should know about using fat-burners for this purpose. One, over time your body will get used to the effects and that "hyper" feeling will disappear unless you cycle off for a couple weeks. Two, not everybody reacts well to ephedrine, a main ingredient which you will also see listed as the herb Ma Huang. Some people get nervous, paranoid, or nauseated when they take ephedrine. Another common side effect is sleeplessness, especially if you take them within five or six hours of going to sleep. I admit that I spent many a sleepless night staring at the ceiling years ago, wondering whether the boost to my training intensity compensated for the lack of sleep I was experiencing as well. Perhaps the worst thing that can happen is that you can become dependent on training on stimulants, and trying to work out without them feels like you're just spinning your wheels. One way that many bodybuilders have dealt with this is to only use stimulants on those days when they train their toughest bodyparts. For instance, if shoulders and arms have never been a problem for you, yet your legs are still a challenge, take them on leg day but not shoulders and arms. Caffeine and ephedrine are actually drugs, they just happen to be legal right now. This means that they can be used to enhance your training, or they can be abused and cause all manner of negative effects. Experiment to find your tolerance level, then be responsible enough to know your limits. You may have seen ads that claim up to 10 % strength increases instantly with these products. I have no vested interests in any of these products, so believe me when I tell you this is no exaggeration. When you're properly 'jacked up' on ephedrine and caffeine, you are definitely able to handle more weight.

Less Frequent Training

Skip LaCour, who I respect deeply as a man, a bodybuilder, and a trusted friend, popularized once-a-week training for bodyparts a few years ago, and it has since been successfully adopted by hundreds of thousands of lifters. It helps motivation and intensity in two ways. For one thing, since the bodypart has a full seven days in which to recover, it is always completely rested and ready to go to war by the time you train it again. Second, because you know you only have that one chance a week to hit that bodypart, a sense of urgency is created that drives you to give that session everything you have. It's also a lot easier to get psyched about training something when it's been a week, rather than if you just trained it only a couple days ago. Finally, because you're only training one part of the body a day, you can get in and out of the gym in under an hour. Here's an example of a split that does this:

Sunday: Off
Monday: Chest
Tuesday: Back
Wednesday: Quads
Thursday: Delts
Friday: Hams and calves
Saturday: Arms

Creating The Right Mental State For Intensity

So far we have addressed everything except what is possibly the most critical component of generating motivation and intensity – your mental state. Call it your attitude, your mood, or what have you, but the results you get from your training will be largely dependent on the state of mind you are in while you work out. You must learn to control your state to optimize performance. First things first. When you're in the gym, you're they're for one reason only, and that's to push your body past its previous limits and force it to respond. This doesn't mean you can't say hello to people or talk to your training partner, but it does mean that you must be all business when it comes time to do your sets. One thing you must never do is talk during your sets. If anyone tries to talk to you, be blunt and say 'no talking.' It's the only way some people will get the point. Unlike you, a lot of men and women aren't in the gym to get results. They might think they are, but the reality is that they wander around and gab it up far more than they exercise. Never let these people suck you into their mediocre ways. If you have to wear headphones in the gym to keep people from bothering you, do it. Your time in the gym is too precious to waste, and you mustn't be distracted from the task at hand.

Next up is the issue of fear. You may be afraid to lift the type of weights you need to if you really want to grow. As long as you warm up with a few minutes of moderate cardio, take two or three progressively heavier warm-ups before launching into your working weight, and employ proper form, your odds for injury are slim. A good training partner who knows how to spot you also helps. You have to take the attitude that you are going to beat the weights, the weights aren't going to beat you.

Now for the really important part. How do you approach your sets so that your mind is primed to tell your body to perform at its absolute peak? You need to come up with your own 'power ritual.' Start watching very strong men in the gym, guys who can bench press more than twice their bodyweight, or squat three times that amount. They are a rare breed, and stand out no matter where they train. Each one of these men has some sort of ritual they go through immediately before attempting a very heavy weight. They might sit with head down and eyes closed, summoning the strength they need from within. They might snap their fingers, breathe rapidly, or even curse to themselves under their breath, snapping themselves into a temporary rage suitable for blasting up a 300-pound military press. Some guys clap their hands together and make a certain grunt or noise that makes them feel unstoppable. Skip LaCour has written extensively about this process. To sum it up, he instructs you to concentrate hard on envisioning a time when you felt strong enough to lift the whole world, then making a gesture he and Anthony Robbins call a 'power move.' The power move can be anything from a karate chop in the air to punching one hand into the other palm. After you go through the reinforcement of the visualization and power move several times, it becomes ingrained. From then on, simply doing the move before your set will put you in the frame of mind or 'state' where you instantly are prepared to do your best. I find that simply breathing faster and talking to myself with encouraging phrases like "come on, got this" is enough to snap me into that state. Staring at myself in the mirror with a decidedly hostile glare serves to magnify this feeling that I am superhuman and capable of lifting any amount of weight I attempt. No doubt, some people will laugh or make fun of you either to your face or behind your back once you start exhibiting this 'strange behavior.' Ignore them. Their acceptance of you isn't going to do a damn thing to help you reach your goals. People are afraid, downright intimidated by such displays of raw intensity and energy. It makes them feel insecure because they never try this hard. That's the basic reason that they never make any progress, and trying harder is the reason you will improve.

Summary

I hope you have learned that motivation and intensity are two things that must flow from inside you. All the pep talks and screaming in your ear from a trainer or coach might work for a while, but ultimately you aren't going to stick with anything for the long run unless it's very important to you and your own desire is high. If you want to improve your physique so much that it's an aching need on your mind most of the time, then the rest will come from that. Believe in yourself, and never, ever give up no matter what.

Avoiding Overtraining

We're all in a rush to reach our own goals in weight training and bodybuilding. That can be a good thing, because it's this enthusiasm that drives us to do the things other people think of as chores – getting to the gym and training hard regularly, eating nutritious food at frequent intervals, and being constantly on the lookout for anything that may speed up or amplify our results. This enthusiasm can have ill effects, however, if taken to extremes. If training is performed too often or in excess amounts for the body to adequately repair itself from the damage inflicted by intense exercise and recharge the nervous system, a condition known as overtraining occurs. Train hard with weights, and you will grow larger and stronger. Train hard too much or too often with weights, and you not only won't grow any larger or stronger, you could actually become smaller and weaker. And since overtraining also weakens the immune system, illnesses like colds, flu's, and strep throats are also common by-products. It hardly seems fair that you can be so gung-ho about your training and be punished by suffering these unpleasant consequences, but it's probably the most common reason why most trainers don't see the results they should. This course is going to help you determine the best training frequencies and volume to avoid this catabolic condition, as well as offer strategies to employ in your nutrition, supplementation, and rest to make sure that your training does exactly what you want it to do – produce positive, meaningful improvements in your body's performance and appearance. By doing as much as you can to stay in an anabolic state, you'll be sure that you are always moving forward in your efforts, instead of standing still or worse – going backward.

Symptoms Of Overtraining

Most people who are overtrained are in denial, not wanting to believe that they could be in such a situation. We all pride ourselves on being intelligent and diligent about our training, so admitting we are overtrained can seem like admission of failure. Don't be ashamed. Everyone overtrains at one time or another, whether you're fourteen years old and just starting to lift, or a Mr. Olympia contender who's been at this game for over fifteen years. The only crime is in not recognizing the signs and doing something to remedy your situation. Here's what to look for:

Unexplained drop in bodyweight or strength
Trouble sleeping
Lack of energy
Loss in appetite
Decreased sex drive
Drop in enthusiasm to train
Increased resting heart beat (taken upon waking)
Lingering colds, coughs, sore throats and flu's
Nagging injuries and/or joint pain
Lack of any progress in size or strength for months on end
Shaking hands, headaches

These are all signals the body sends to indicate that you are in an overtrained state. Of course, some are also indicative of more serious illnesses and should be evaluated by a doctor if they persist. Should you continue to ignore these signs, chances are that your body will do something drastic to force you to stop training altogether. In extreme cases, major injuries such as muscle tears, and crippling illnesses like pneumonia and mononucleosis have resulted from athletes continuing to push their bodies too hard for too long without heeding the danger signs. What's more relevant to most of you is that in an overtrained condition, gains just don't materialize. None of us want to spin our wheels, busting our asses with the weights for nothing in return. But that's exactly what's happening to untold thousands of lifters right now. You may be one of them, or you may simply want to avoid becoming one of them. Let's educate you on how to stay out of this mess.

Training issues

How Often Should You Train?

The main culprit in overtraining is working out too often. What constitutes too often is an individual matter. We all have various levels of recovery ability, which is nothing more than our body's ability to regenerate itself and be ready to train again. This doesn't only pertain to the muscles themselves, but also the central nervous system. While you may not be interfering with the recovery of your chest by training legs the following day, you are still heavily taxing the nervous system any time you work out with high intensity. Some of us can train five or six days a week without overly taxing the nervous system. For others, anything more than three non-consecutive days, such as a Monday-Wednesday-Friday program, would start frazzling them out. Often those who have trained at a high level for sports that demanded almost daily practice have nervous systems that are adapted to training more frequently without ill effects.

What about how many days in a row you should train? Most drug-free lifters are safe to train two days in a row, but three starts to push it. A two-on, one-off schedule like this is about right for the majority:

Two-on, One off	
Day one:	Back
Day two:	Shoulders and triceps
Day three:	Rest
Day four:	Legs
Day five:	Chest and biceps
Day six:	Rest
REPEAT CYCLE	

Some trainers work out more frequently, but only hit one bodypart a day, as popularized by Team Universe and Musclemania Champion Skip LaCour.

Six-on, One off	
Sunday:	Back
Monday:	Chest
Tuesday:	Quads
Wednesday:	Shoulders
Thursday:	Hams and calves
Friday:	Arms
Saturday:	Rest

Although this may seem like more training, the sessions are shorter. For everything except perhaps back, you should be able to complete the workout in 45 minutes or less. Also, each bodypart has a full seven days to recover. If your nervous system just can't handle going to the gym without a full day of rest afterward, try this:

Every Other Day	
Day one:	Chest and biceps
Day two:	Rest
Day three:	Back and triceps
Day four:	Rest
Day five:	Legs
Day six:	Rest
Day seven:	Shoulders, calves, abs
Day eight:	Rest
REPEAT CYCLE	

Or, if you want to take the weekends off to recover and recharge more fully, try three days a week.

Three Days A Week	
Sunday:	Rest
Monday:	Back and biceps
Tuesday:	Rest
Wednesday:	Chest, shoulders, triceps
Thursday:	Rest
Friday:	Legs
Saturday:	Rest

These are some good frequencies to try. Experiment for two weeks with each if you are unsure, and make a note of your energy levels and enthusiasm as you evaluate which one seems to work best for you.

How Many Sets?

The amount of sets you can tolerate and still respond to positively also depends on the individual, but if you are working in the standard rep ranges of 8-12 for the upper body and 12-20 for the lower, you probably never need to do more than three or at most four work sets for any one exercise. If you can't exhaust the muscle with four sets of any given exercise (taking each set to failure), either you aren't training hard enough or you have incredible muscle endurance. You also don't want to do too many exercises for any one bodypart. Here are some general guidelines as to the correct number of sets for various muscle groups, based on average trainers with normal recovery ability. None of these include warm-up sets.

Chest:	8-12 Sets
Back:	10-16 sets
Legs:	10-16 sets
Shoulders:	8-12 sets
Biceps:	6-9 sets
Triceps:	9-12 sets
Calves:	4-6 sets

I am sure you have read many routines of the pro's which list sets far in excess of these amounts, which I will explain away shortly. For the average, drug-free trainer, these are the ranges which will foster results and at the same time prevent overtraining.

Heavy Duty

The late Mike Mentzer believed that most of us actually have even far less recovery ability than commonly thought, and that subsequently nearly all lifters are overtrained. His prescriptions for training frequency and volume grew more curtailed by the year. By the last couple years of his life, he was advocating training no more than once every five or six days, for just one all-out set of five or six exercises. I doubt that many people in the world are actually so "recovery-challenged" as to require this much rest, and I further contend that it would be impossible for most people to make any progress on such a system. If the muscles are not trained very soon after they are fully recovered, they actually begin to 'de-train,' or lose size and strength. Nonetheless, it is only fair to acknowledge that there are those rare individuals for whom this style of training is necessary. They tend to be extreme ectomorphs (naturally tall and skinny) with very fast metabolisms, and possess nervous or 'high-strung' personalities. Having demanding, high-stress jobs and multiple responsibilities also improves your chances of falling into Mr. Mentzer's category. If you need as much rest and recovery as Heavy Duty dictates, here is an example of the type of training it entails. Remember, only one all-out set of each exercise is performed, after your warm-ups.

	Squat
	Bench press
Routine A	Barbell row
	Military press
	Barbell curl
Rest four full days, then:	
	Deadlift
	Chin
Routine B	Pec Dec
	Lateral Raise
	Weighted dip
Rest four full days, then repeat sequence	

Avoiding Exercise Redundancy

A major contributing factor to overtraining that many lifters are unaware of is redundancy in exercise selection. They will waste valuable energy performing several exercises that work the muscle in nearly the exact same way. You often see someone doing the following type of routine for their chest:

Barbell bench press	3 x 8-12
Flat dumbbell press	3 x 8-12
Hammer Strength machine flat press	3 x 8-12
Flat dumbbell flyes	3 x 8-12
Pec dec	3 x 8-12
Incline dumbbell press	3 x 8-12
Incline Smith Machine press	3 x 8-12

What's wrong with this workout, besides 21 sets being almost twice as many as most people need for their chests? The first three exercises were all basically the same, as were the next two and the last two. This person did seven exercises for their chest, when they should have only done three. Without a basic foundation of exercise physiology, it's easy to fall into similar traps. Many people will perform squats, leg presses, and hack squats in a single leg-training session, not realizing that all pressing movements for the legs are essentially the same exercise. We all want to 'cover all the angles' and make certain that the muscle has been worked properly. This list will help you accomplish this goal economically, so that you don't waste valuable time and energy in your workouts.

Quadriceps	a leg extension, any pressing movement (squats, leg press, etc)
Hamstrings	a leg curl, a stiff-leg deadlift
Back:	a row, a chin, a shrug, and a lower back movement such as hyperextensions or good mornings. Deadlifts are also advised for those seeking maximum mass and power in the back.
Chest:	a flat or decline press, a flye movement, an incline press
Shoulders:	an overhead press, a side lateral movement, a rear lateral movement
Biceps:	any palms-up curl, and any reverse or hammer grip curl
Triceps:	any extension, plus either dips or close-grip bench press
Calves:	standing or donkey calf raise, and seated calf raise
Abs:	any exercise that brings the knees to the torso, and any exercise that brings the torso to the knees

Anything beyond these is usually unnecessary overkill, and puts you in danger of overtraining. As 8-time Mr. Olympia Lee Haney said, "Stimulate, don't annihilate!"

What About Cardio?

Cardio is a tricky subject. Because it is in fact additional exercise, it does indeed make increased demands on your recovery ability. Without it, though, most of us start accumulating more bodyfat than we would like. Experiment to find your acceptable limits. Start with three weekly sessions of twenty minutes each, either on the days you train (after your weight training, not before) or on your off days. If you seem to be able to handle it without running into any of the symptoms of overtraining, you can increase it until your bodyfat levels are acceptable. It does seem, however, that sessions longer than 35-45 minutes begin to take you into a catabolic zone, even under the best of conditions. It must be said that some people with more limited recovery abilities can't tolerate any amount of cardio on top of their weight training without edging into overtraining. Luckily, most of these individuals tend to be naturally lean anyway. In summary, pay close attention to how much cardio you do, as excessive cardio can definitely make you more likely to be overtrained.

The Effects Of Steroids, And Why The Pro's Routines Aren't For Drug-free Lifters

Some of you who haven't been around bodybuilding very long may not yet realize that the majority of top amateur and professional bodybuilders depend heavily on steroids. This is the main reason why they are able to train more frequently and with far more exercises and sets. Steroids are very powerful drugs that allow users to work harder and longer. They also greatly accelerate the recovery process, so steroid users can train more often without the risk of overtraining. Pro's will often train the entire body in sections over three or four consecutive days before taking a day off, and rarely exhibit any symptoms of overtraining. They can also get away with performing as many as twice the number of sets recommended above for bodyparts with similar impunity. Most of the readers of physique publications like *Flex* and *Muscle and Fitness* who attempt to follow the routines of the pro's wind up overtrained instead of growing. Because steroid use is a felony, the athletes and magazines can't really tell you all these truths without risk of legal problems. Nobody wants to get in that kind of trouble. Of course, you can easily avoid overtraining without drugs by following the protocols we are discussing herein. Steroids simply allow you to avoid overtraining without paying attention to all these factors.

Nutritional Methods For Recovery

John Parrillo, one of the industry's top experts in training and nutrition, has a famous quote: "There's no such thing as overtraining – only undereating." While there obviously is such a phenomenon as overtraining, he has a valid point in that most lifters don't eat enough of the right foods at the right times to keep the recovery process moving along smoothly at all times. Most trainers drastically underestimate their own nutritional needs. Here is what you need to know in more concise terms.

You must eat 1-2 grams of high-quality protein per pound of bodyweight a day. Without this amount, the systems of the body will not have the raw materials from which to repair the muscle tissue damaged by high-intensity training and supercompensate (restore them slightly bigger and stronger than before as an adaptation mechanism). This is best accomplished over the course of 5-7 daily meals, which should be a mix of solid meals and shakes or bars. The main goal is to always be in an anabolic, or building state. To avoid falling into a catabolic, or wasting state, you must not allow yourself to ever experience the sensation of strong hunger. Within 2-3 hours of a solid meal, the food has been digested and it's time to get another meal or shake in. A shake will only hold you for an hour, and a bar for 60-90 minutes. It may sound like you are being asked to make eating a full-time job – you are! It's a big commitment, but this is what it takes to keep your muscles 'well-fed.' A starving muscle is a shrinking muscle, unfortunately. A particularly important time to get a shake down is immediately after training, as this is when your body is totally depleted of amino acids and glycogen. You want a shake that can be digested as quickly as possible to jumpstart the recovery process. Current studies show that a mix of 30-50 grams of whey protein and a mix of 50-70 grams of maltodextrin and simple sugars is best for meeting these unique needs. Getting another meal in within an hour with a similar 1-3 ratio of protein and carbs (either another shake or a solid meal) is also imperative to 'refill your tanks.' If you don't get the nutrients in inside this brief window of opportunity, your ability to recover for your next session will be severely compromised. If you have never had a shake like this after training, you will be amazed at how fast you go from feeling wiped out to energized again. Carbs in general are needed most in the meal before you train (especially slower-burning carbs like rice or oatmeal that deliver a more sustained energy flow) and in the meals within the two hours after you finish training. Don't be afraid to eat more unless you begin to gain excess fat.

Essential fatty acids are also needed to facilitate the muscle recovery and building process. You can either take two tablespoons of flax seed oil every day, or take your fats in the form of omega-3 or evening primrose oil capsules. Reasonable amounts of dietary fat in the form of whole eggs and red meat are also beneficial.

A final time to get more protein in that most people overlook is while you are sleeping. Keep a container in your refrigerator with a pre-mixed shake that should be either 100% casein (a slow-burning milk protein) or a blend of casein and whey. Eight hours is too long to go without protein for hard-training athletes such as bodybuilders and serious weight trainers. Whenever you get up to urinate, drink your shake. If you know you usually get up more than once, try to ration out about 20-30 grams at a time. If you don't usually get up to urinate, try drinking a glass of water right before retiring. That should wake you up within a few hours. I don't recommend setting an alarm, as this disrupts your natural sleep patterns. You may find it hard to go back to sleep after being awoken by an alarm, and losing sleep is not conducive to staying anabolic in the least.

Eat well and eat often so that your muscles always have a steady stream of nutrients available.

Supplements For Recovery

There are several supplements that bodybuilders and strength athletes use to enhance recovery. The shake we discussed after training is a key ingredient, as is the amino acid L-Glutamine. L-Glutamine has been shown to boost the immune system and speed up the body's own regeneration process. It is sold in powder form or in capsules. Twenty grams a day are recommended on training days, ten either mixed in or with your post-workout shake, and another ten before bedtime. On non-training days, take ten grams before bedtime only. Another supplement that shows promise is the cortisol-blocker phosphatidylserine, or PS for short. Cortisol is the stress hormone released in response to various stressful situations – weight training being one of them. It is responsible for many of the wasting effects that often occur from intense physical exertion. Ever wonder why a lot of men lose up to twenty pounds during military boot camp, even if they didn't have any fat to lose in the first place? In essence, cortisol signals the body to break down the amino acids inside your muscles for fuel – literally eating your muscles away. PS isn't 100% proven yet to be effective, but if you can spare the extra expense, it's a pretty good insurance policy second to L-Glutamine. And of course, protein powder can be considered a supplement to enhance recovery, as staying in a positive nitrogen balance at all times is essential to remaining anabolic. Finally, anti-oxidant multi-vitamins may also be helpful. Since they combat the effects of free-radical damage due to environmental factors such as air pollution, they could theoretically assist in clearing the waste products from training out of the muscles at a faster rate as well.

Sleep And Rest

I'm sure you already know that you require eight hours of sleep a night. Unfortunately, many of us don't get those eight hours, especially if we have demanding jobs and families to care for. Try to reach this figure somehow, even if it means sneaking a few 15-minute naps a day whenever you can. It will be difficult at first to relax and fall asleep so quickly, but you will adapt in time. Nearly every MD learns how to master the art of the opportune nap in their residency phase, when shifts can run as long as 48 hours straight. If you have to wait until the weekend or a day off, try to make up for the lost sleep then. If you fail to meet the basic requirements of sleep, both your recovery ability and immune function will be compromised. If you are able to get nine or ten hours of sleep a day, even better. Flex Wheeler confided to me that he actually made his best progress in his final two years of an amateur when he was able to sleep 12-16 hours a day! In that time, he grew from one of the smallest heavyweights on the national scene to a dominant heavyweight who won the '92 USA decisively, then went on to win his first two professional contests. There is no doubt that all that sleep was a major factor in his success. I realize that almost no one has this much free time to be catching z's, but take advantage whenever you do. For example, there's no reason to be staying up late watching TV instead of going to bed early. Those couple hours could make the difference for you between recovering and not recovering.

Also, try to avoid any extra physical activity beyond your training. If it sounds like I'm telling you to be lazy, I am. Anything else you do, such as playing basketball, riding your mountain bike, or a game of football in the park with your buddies, cuts into your limited amount of energy and recovery ability. Many teenagers have problems gaining weight because they are so physically active in other areas. A physical job such as construction or package delivery will also make it harder to avoid overtraining. If you have a choice and the money is the same, go for a desk job or at least one that doesn't make excessive physical demands on your body. But overtraining affects at least half the population of serious lifters at any given moment. Getting enough sleep and rest will go a long way toward keeping you out of that quagmire.

Reducing Stress

We briefly touched on cortisol's destructive role, but understand that any type of stress can result in the release of this nasty hormone. If you are the type of person who worries all the time or goes off the handle every time someone cuts you off in traffic, you owe it to yourself to try to learn to relax and take things in stride. Go with the flow. Never let yourself get all worked up over situations that you have no control over. Say you get a speeding ticket or are involved in a car accident. It's easy to let either event consume you in anger and frustration, but this will release a flood of cortisol. Try to see things in a larger perspective. If you have a ticket, that's it. Accept that you will either pay it or fight it, but either way getting angry and stressed out isn't going to change the outcome. What's done is done. There are many books and audiocassettes available on stress management and relaxation. If you find yourself unable to control your temper or your stress levels, consider them a worthy investment not only to improve your life in general, but especially your bodybuilding. The more serene and calm you can remain, except for the hellish intensity of your training, of course, the better equipped your body will be to rebuild itself and grow.

Layoffs

The last issue to address in order to avoid overtraining is taking occasional time off from training. For some of you, this will be even harder than eating all the meals and getting enough sleep. We all want to achieve our results as fast as we can, and missing workouts hardly seems conducive to that end. Of course, the contrary is actually true. Our bodies simply can't take the constant pounding and abuse of heavy weight training indefinitely without a break every now and then. Most experts recommend taking a full week off for every 8-16 weeks of training. Where you fall on that scale depends on how easily you tend to overtrain. This week off does several important things. It gives your entire body, not only your muscles but also your connective tissues and nervous system, some much-needed rest. Rather than come back weaker a week later, you'll probably find yourself actually feeling stronger and more energetic. Layoffs are also crucial from a mental perspective. I don't care how motivated you are about training, I don't know anyone who can stay psyched about lifting forever. Let's face it – training by its very nature is a repetitive activity. Not necessarily boring, that it should never be, but definitely repetitive. By forcibly removing yourself from the gym for a week or ten days, you recharge your enthusiasm. By the time you do return to training, you're so raring to go that you will practically tear the gym apart, melt it down with white-hot intensity. Many people find themselves breaking through plateaus shortly after layoffs, reaching levels of size and strength that probably wouldn't have even been possible without the break. I recently took nearly two weeks off of training while my family and I vacationed in Cancun. It was the longest break from training I had experienced since the mid-1980's. Did I look forward to lifting again? Let's just say I was practically shaking with anticipation when I finally returned to the gym. That's the magic of layoffs. Not only are they an essential component of avoiding the overtraining syndrome, but they will keep you from getting stuck in physical and mental ruts.

Summary

Overtraining is a very real problem for anyone who is trying to improve his or her body through weight training. There is a fine line between training enough to stimulate gains, and training so much that no gains are allowed to materialize. Follow the advice I have given you here, and you should always be on the right side of the fence – the side where you grow! Best of luck to you.

Safety – Yes, You Can Get Hurt

Many parents worry about their kids lifting weights, because they don't want them to get hurt. And to be honest, that concern is justified, since you can indeed incur injuries ranging from minor to severe. Most injuries happen for two reasons; bad form and using too much weight. Usually those two factors go hand in hand, and young men are especially prone to these training transgressions. It's all about that macho attitude and sense of invincibility that accompany that flood of natural testosterone in a developing male's body. I was only eighteen when my own youthful bravado took me out of training commission for the first time.

My first two training injuries happened almost back-to-back. I popped my cherry while doing overhead presses, seated on a flat bench with no back support. I was using an EZ-curl bar and alternating reps of pressing to the front and back. Don't ask me where I learned that one, I have no recollection. Even then I used to train to failure, meaning until I could no longer budge the bar. Depending on which rep I failed at, I would get stuck with the bar either on my neck or across my clavicles. This time it happened to be the back of my neck. To get it off me, I had to somehow push up another half-rep to clear it over my big melon head. This involved a spastic burst of the torso as I essentially ducked under the weight and transferred it in front of me. In the act of doing this, I felt something snap in my lower back like a rubber band. Having never had a lower back injury yet in my life, I was in a panic as the pain set in. It wasn't too bad at first, actually, just really tight and sore. By the next morning I was in a whole new world of pain. Just putting on my socks, jeans, and sneakers was an arduous, agonizing process. I had to wear my leather weight belt cinched tightly under my denim jacket to keep my spine straight, as any bending at all sent shooting pains up and down its length. Luckily I was a college student at UCSB and the student clinic was free, but the doctor was both unhelpful and unsympathetic. "Welcome to back pain, most Americans suffer it at some point," he told me dryly.

"What should I do about it?" His eyes glanced down at the Gold's Gym logo on my T-shirt (at 5-8 and 145 pounds, it was my only way of telling the world I was a muscle man in the making) and frowned with disapproval.

"Stop lifting weights." Over seventeen years have passed since that day in the clinic, but I still feel I owe that guy the middle finger and a hearty "Fuck you" for his lack of compassion.

That was my first of what would be dozens of lower back injuries. My first shoulder injury happened not two weeks later – apparently I was on a roll. This time it was on the one true marker of not only a young man's strength, but his manhood as well – the barbell bench press. For the past year and a half I had been maxing out on this lift, seeking greater and greater numbers. I had no plan, assuming that if I just kept pushing harder and harder I would get stronger. The problem was that I never recognized how badly I was cheating. First of all, I always needed a spotter. This was not so much for safety as for having someone to lift part of the weight for me, though I was never consciously aware of this foolish idea. On the night I hurt my shoulder, I was attempting to bench press 275 pounds, which was probably about 50 pounds more than I could actually bench press for one rep. I was doing my usual tricks; arching my back like crazy, wiggling my hips, and using the worst possible body mechanics. This injury was sudden and unexpected too. As I was bouncing the weight off my chest (yet another smart move), something tore inside my left shoulder, most likely my rotator cuff.

Bad form was to blame in both cases.

Most Common Weight Training Injuries

Talk to anyone who has been training for a few years or longer, and they will almost always have more than one injury to report. Shoulders are a very common problem area, as are knees, lower back, and elbows. The most dramatic injuries are muscle tears. When IFBB pro Jean-Pierre Fux tore both his quads during a photo shoot with Chris Lund for *Flex* magazine, the series of photos from the incident were shown over and over again. I also recall when Kevin Levrone tore his pec in 1993, every magazine had photos of his torso, stained purple with internal bleeding and bruising in a huge pool around the injury, extending out to his biceps. But muscle tears are not something that happens to most bodybuilders, and it seems that the biggest man are in the highest-risk group. The reason for this is that the muscles have a great deal of potential to become bigger and stronger, while the tendons and ligaments do not. When the muscles grow to enormous dimensions, as you see in pro bodybuilders that commonly weigh 250-300 pounds at under six feet tall, the connective tissues only grow a small amount in relation to them. Thus, if substantial force is generated, the muscle can easily tear off the joint or bone.

Far more common are strains and pulls, which are merely words to describe partial tears. Usually these partial tears will heal on their own if the area is left alone for a few weeks. Of course, bodybuilders having the mentality that we do, often these partial tears are either totally ignored or not given enough time to heal before training the area again, and we either re-injure it or tear it worse than before.

The most common injuries of all are simple 'wear and tear' injuries from overuse. Personally, I don't think the human body was meant to lift very heavy weights day after day for periods of many years. The shoulder, knee, and elbow joints take a real beating from the best mass-building exercises like bench presses, squats, overhead presses, deadlifts, dips, barbell extensions, and so on. The guys who train the heaviest seem to rack up the most injuries, on average. As many bodybuilders age and accumulate injuries, they are often forced to abandon many movements that cause them joint pain. Ironically, they often find they are able to retain their mass or even continue to make gains with different exercises, or simply by using less weight and concentrating more on the contraction and the pump. In my case, I suffer from such severe tendonitis in the left elbow where the triceps attach to the joint that I have been unable to perform any type of extension movement, with the exception of dumbbell kickbacks, for at least five years now. Even using light weight on exercises like skull crushers or overhead extensions is agonizing. However, I have continued to train heavy on various extension movements with cables, and my triceps are certainly much larger than they were five years ago.

So, finding exercise that don't aggravate an injury or joint pain is one way to extend your training career and keep gaining. Another is to rotate exercises on a regular basis. Overuse happens because we do the same exact movements again and again. If you do bench presses with a bar sometimes, with dumbbells at other times, and at still other times with something like a Hammer Strength machine, you decrease your risk of developing the nagging overuse injuries that have plagued millions of long-term weight trainers over the years. But I still feel very strongly that the very best way to prevent injuries of all kinds is to use proper form.

Where Do We Learn Proper Form?

Monkey see, monkey do. That time-worn cliché explains why most men and women don't know how to perform exercises correctly. Most people don't hire good personal trainers to start them out right, so they just imitate what they see others in the gym doing. Another obstacle men have to deal with is our own machismo. Like fixing cars and playing football, lifting weights is something all men are supposed to know how to do. To admit that you don't know how is to concede that you aren't a 'real man.' It's almost as bad as stopping to ask for directions when you're lost! So, rather than seek out someone that actually knows how to do exercises the right way with proper body mechanics, most males prefer to flounder in ignorance, assuming that it doesn't really matter how you lift the weight anyway, as long as you lift it and use as much weight as you can.

In the old days, you could excuse this ignorance. There was no Internet, bodybuilding magazines were hard to come by, and personal trainers were as rare as albinos. Form was passed on by older brothers, football coaches, friends, or mimicked at the gym. Fast-forward to the present day, and solid information is a lot easier to find for those who seek it. There are a plethora of bodybuilding web sites loaded with articles on training. Some, like www.bodybuilding.com, even have video clips demonstrating proper form in detail. Every month, magazines are loaded with illustrated training articles, and instructional DVD's and CD-ROMs are abundant. There are now hundreds of thousands of certified personal trainers in the USA alone. True, not all are as experienced and knowledgeable, but there are still plenty that are. I tend to favor those with a bodybuilding background, if a bodybuilding type of physique is what you desire for yourself. Most of us don't have the type of discretionary income to hire a trainer for the long term, but it's still a good idea to at least enlist the services of one for five to ten sessions, until the basics of good form on most exercises are mastered. True mastery of form only comes with time, and has a great deal to do with developing a strong mind-muscle connection. Two men may appear to the casual observer to be using equally good form, but the man with superior mind-muscle connection will always be doing a better job of stimulating the target muscle.

Wear And Tear Of Heavy Training Over Time

Even with proper form, it's almost guaranteed that if you train long enough, you will have chronic aches and pains in areas like the lower back, shoulders, elbows, and knees. These are overuse injuries, the result of pounding heavy weights week after week, year after year. You can avoid this to some extent by taking regular layoffs from training, as well as alternating heavy and light days, or intentionally scheduling heavier and lighter training periods. But rare is the man that trains heavy for any length of time and doesn't have some type of battle scar. It's why a lot of men in their thirties, forties, and fifties tend to shy away from certain exercises that aggravate these injured or chronically painful areas. For instance, my elbows are chronically inflamed, and any type of extension movement for the triceps with free weights has been impossible for me since about 2000. I train around the injury by using cables and emphasizing weighted dips or dip machines, rather than relying on skull crushers or overhead dumbbell extensions. Due to lower back or knee injuries, some men can't squat anymore, and substitute the leg press. Machines can get the job done, too. The Hammer Strength line is particularly popular and effective. I still believe that the free weight basics belong in your routine if you can do them, but if you can't, there's no need to abandon training altogether when you have options.

Veteran lifters also often employ physical therapy, massage therapy, and chiropractic treatments in an attempt to continue hard training as they age. In extreme cases, orthopedic surgeons may need to intervene when injuries are severe. But the good news is that such surgery has become quite advanced in recent years. For instance, many times a man gets his knee 'scoped,' or has arthroscopic surgery performed, and is up and walking the same day, and back to light cardio and leg training in just a couple weeks.

This chapter has probably been the most important one, because as far as I am concerned, real bodybuilding is all about the training. To get results, and to keep getting results, you need to train both hard and smart.

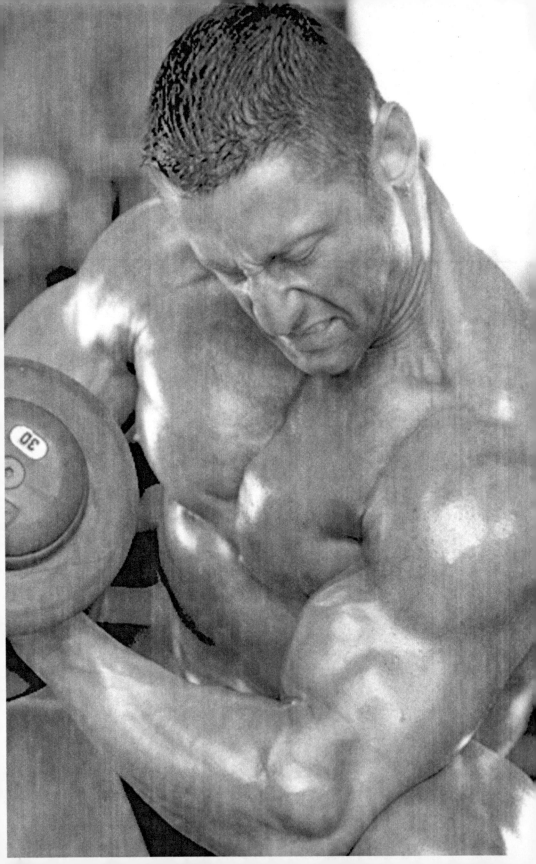

05

NUTRITION – HOW TO EAT TO GAIN MUSCLE AND LOSE FAT

Eating To Gain Weight

Now we move on to the second side of the triangle, your nutrition. The main idea to keep in mind about nutrition is that your body needs a steady stream of nutrients to recover from the damage inflicted to your muscles by your training and to support new muscle growth. You need quality food at frequent intervals. Depending on the fat content of the meal, two to four hours is how long it is going to take your food to digest. A low-fat meal such as a grilled chicken breast, a bowl of rice, and some broccoli will be digested in two hours or so. Pizza or barbecued ribs, which contain a great deal of fat, will take closer to four hours. Liquid meals like protein or meal-replacement shakes will clear your stomach in an hour, while supplement bars take 60-90 minutes. If you are eating mostly low-fat fare and throw a couple shakes in, you should be able to fit in six or seven meals while awake. One thing you never want to feel is hunger pangs in your stomach. Once you do, you can rest assured that your body is now venturing into a catabolic state where your own muscles are in danger of being robbed of their amino acids for fuel. Thus, you are better off feeling full or stuffed than you are experiencing hunger. This is a case where having a bit extra in your system is superior to not having enough. If gaining weight has been a real struggle for you, odds are your caloric intake has not been sufficient to meet the needs of your metabolism and energy output.

Appetite

Some people genuinely don't have very large appetites, and forcing down the amount of food that they need to grow makes them gag. If you're one of those types who gets full very quickly, you must treat your eating like your weight training. You don't go from benching 100 pounds to 400 pounds in a month, and you shouldn't attempt to increase your daily calories from 1,500 to 5,000 in a month, either. (There are free calorie counters all over the Internet, or you can get a book like *The Calorie Bible* to use as a reference.) Gradually try to eat just a little more each day, and your body will slowly grow accustomed to larger volumes of food. Another trick that those with small appetites employ is to eat as much solid food as they can at a sitting, then top it off with a shake to add more nutrients. Even when you're full, you can still manage to swallow a few gulps of liquid. You will also find that regular exercise stimulates your appetite, so you should see a marked increase in your eating capacity if you haven't been training consistently.

Can I Gain Pure Muscle With No Fat?

Certain people can indeed gain muscle at an appreciable rate without accumulating any added bodyfat. The majority of these people are using steroids, are teenagers with naturally high testosterone and GH levels, or are genetically predisposed to such a favorable ratio of gains (most 'easy gainers' put on muscle exclusively). Most of us have to put on a little bit of fat to gain a lot of muscle. The rationale is that those seeking to gain weight must be sure to always be in a state of caloric surplus, not in caloric deficit or even maintaining. To be absolutely sure that you are taking in enough protein and calories, it is wise to err on the side of caution and take in a bit more than what you may actually need. Of course, if you find yourself gaining a large amount of fat, you have obviously gone overboard and need to scale back your intake. For years this practice of taking in excess nutrients has been known as "bulking up," and it has worked perfectly for generations of lifters. The extra calories and fat allow the use of heavier weights, which in turn leads to better gains. Once the desired gains have been made, you can trim off the fat to reveal all the new muscle below.

Competitive bodybuilders the world over follow this cycle of bulking up and trimming down. Dorian Yates, for example, used to bulk up to about 310 pounds in the off-season, yet every time he dieted down he proved he had built new muscle in the process. Lee Priest is another proponent of bulking up. Lee started competing internationally as an amateur lightweight in his teenage years, under 154 pounds, but thanks to nearly fifteen seasons of bulking up to lift heavier, he now competes at over 220. The bottom line is that yes, you will have to gain a little fat along with your muscle. The good news is that it doesn't have to be an excessive amount, and you can diet it off whenever you're ready. Now let's look at the macronutrients your meals will be built from.

Protein – The Main Ingredient To Muscle

The most important aspect of eating for gains is taking in enough protein. How much is enough has been up for debate for many years, but the accepted ranges fall between one and two grams per pound of bodyweight a day. I tend to lean more toward two grams. The best sources for protein are eggs, milk, chicken, fish, cottage cheese, steak, ground meat, and turkey. All of these are complete proteins, meaning they contain all of the essential amino acids. Vegetable proteins like nuts, beans, soy milk and tofu are incomplete, lacking several of the key aminos. All of your meals should contain a serving of quality protein. To arrive at how much you should be taking in at each meal, simply do a little math. If you weigh 150 pounds and want to take in two grams per pound of bodyweight, that's 300 grams a day. If you figure out that you can eat six times a day, that works out to fifty grams at each serving. Fifty grams is about two chicken breasts, seven whole eggs, or a can and 2/3 of tuna. Whatever happens, make sure you always get your protein in every two to four hours. If you can cut it closer to two, I would do it. Protein gives you the building blocks that your body uses to grow new muscle tissue, and without it you're screwed. Never forget about getting your protein, and never blow it off. You need it to grow, simple as that. A diet that is deficient in protein will make it nearly impossible to grow any new muscle tissue. I think that's reason enough to justify devoting your attention every day to ensure you take enough in.

Carbs – The Energy Source For Your Muscles

Carbs have a bad reputation lately, largely due to the popularity of the Atkins Diet, which I personally believe to be a gimmick and impossible to maintain forever. Eating more carbs than your body needs will indeed lead to the surplus contributing to bodyfat gains. That much is true. However, the carbs you will be consuming on my nutrition plan will not be simple sugars like bread, bagels, candy, fruit juice, or potato chips. This is the type of carbohydrate that most obese people eat in excess. When you combine inactivity with an orgy of simple carbs and fat, you get a lot of fat. When you combine heavy, intense weight training with complex carbs like rice, yams, oatmeal, and oatmeal, you get a lot of muscle (assuming you are taking in enough protein). Also, carbs have a 'protein-sparing' effect. When you eat more complex carbs, which converts to glucose in the body, you can get away with eating a bit less protein and not risk catabolism. Glucose in turn converts to glucagon, which is stored in the liver. This is what fuels anaerobic exercise, which uses ATP (adenosine triphosphate) production as its fuel source. The two types of chemical reactions that produce ATP are anaerobic glycolysis and the creatine phosphate system. Our body can also use a fatty metabolism by-product called ketone bodies as fuel, but carbs are most definitely the preferred source. To really take this down to "bodybuilding nutrition for Dummies" terms for the hell of it, without eating sufficient carbs at the right times, you will neither have the energy to sustain a productive workout nor the necessary nutrients to replace what was lost, thus sabotaging the results of whatever was accomplished in the gym. And, if weight gain is your sincere gain, you need carbs for their clean but substantial caloric content as well. To put it in folksy terms, complex carbs 'stick to your ribs' rather than sit in your stomach like a pizza, a couple cheeseburgers, or a big hunk of birthday cake does. Fibrous carbs are vegetables like broccoli, carrots, lettuce, cauliflower, green beans, and cucumbers. They are more useful for nutrition plans to get lean, but you still need them for their vitamins, minerals, and ability to keep your digestive tract clean and running smoothly. That's pretty damn important when you eat five to seven meals a day.

Carbs Before Training

For excellent workouts, you need to be sure you 'carb up' before any training session. How soon depends on how whether or not you combined your carbs with protein, particularly solid meat proteins like chicken, steak, or tuna. If you do, wait 90-120 minutes from the time you finish eating until you start your workout. Complex carbs take about an hour to digest when eaten alone (the simplest carbs, like fruit and fruit juice, take only 15-30 minutes). Eating them in combination with solid protein slows the digestive process down to two hours. A shake will not slow down the one-hour mark to any large degree. If you train first thing in the morning, as I do, you would want to wake up and eat something like a bowl of oatmeal or cream of wheat with a protein shake. That way you can train in an hour. Some people try to eat fruit or fruit juice instead as they can be both eaten and digested faster, but then you have to deal with the giant insulin rush and subsequent crash in blood sugar levels. Try to have a great workout when you're yawning and feel like curling up to a nice comfy bench for a nap! If you train after a standard 8-9 hour workday, you will want to have some carbs for lunch, and another serving at the correct point preceding your workout. If you ate some rice or potatoes with lunch at one P.M. and won't be hitting the gym floor until six P.M, try to have some complex carbs sometime around four-thirty or five, preferably with a protein shake. If you are able to have another solid meal in there at some point with meat or fish, try to get that finished 90-120 minutes before you start training. During my best period of gaining muscle, 1989-1994, I felt my best workouts were the ones which came at the end of a day where I had eaten several servings of complex carbs. My tank was always more than full enough to use some very heavy weights over fairly long workouts without running out of steam. Whether you only get one serving in before your workout or six, make sure you don't skimp on the complex carbs.

Carbs After Training

The time immediately after you finish your workout is a very narrow window of opportunity. The reason is that this is the very beginning of the critical recovery and regeneration process. Your body is like a sponge at this moment, possessing a temporarily enhanced ability to absorb certain key nutrients like glucose and amino acids. Take advantage of this fleeting condition, and you will substantially accelerate the recovery process so that super-compensation (i.e. muscle growth) can occur before you subject your body to further punishment in the gym. Ignore this golden moment to replenish lost nutrients, and you will short-circuit the recovery process. You heard that right. Without putting back carbs and protein after weight training, you will not totally recover for your next workout. You also want to consume these carbs and protein in a rapidly digested form. The best choice is a shake containing whey protein hydrolysates and maltodextrin, a medium-chain carbohydrate made from corn. As I write this, more supplement companies are adding simple sugars like dextrose for the resulting insulin spike, which theoretically increases the speed of absorption. The shake should fulfill your numerical requirement for each meal, plus double the grams of total carbs. This shake must be drank as soon as possible after you finish training. Some people think it's okay to wait until they get home, anywhere from 15-45 minutes, to have the shake. I firmly believe the longer you wait, the more you lose out on that opportunity to put your recovery in high gear. Either bring a pre-mixed shake with you in a cooler, buy one at the gym's juice bar if it has one, or bring a container and powder to mix up with water as soon as you're done. Next, between 60-90 minutes later, eat a solid meal with that same ratio of protein to carbs, but only complex carbs this time. Never ignore this crucial need for carbs in the hours after training. It is a vital component to the success of your weight-gain program.

Carbs At Other Times

Feel free to have both starchy (complex) and fibrous carbs with all your meals, if you so desire. In fact, eat as much as you want. Should you start gaining more fat than you are comfortable with, simply cut back on the carbs, though not in the meal before your training and the hours following it.

Fats – Essential For Health And Performance

Dietary fats, like carbs, have a bad reputation for contributing to bodyfat stores, and with good reason. Fatty foods like pizza, pastries, pork, potato and corn chips, and fried chicken are the weapon of choice for America's obese. Eating a lot of fat, more so when combined with carbs, is a guaranteed way to get very fat yourself. The thing is, our body needs certain essential fatty acids for many key functions. Many of these functions are related to anabolism, so eating a very low-fat diet will also impede muscle gains. These days some guys are getting their fats from a couple daily tablespoons of flax seed oil instead of eating a brick of cheese, a rack of barbecued ribs, or a double cheeseburger. You might have such a fast metabolism that you can eat substantial amounts of saturated fat every day without getting fat or having problems with high cholesterol. There are people like that out there. I have seen them. Then again, you might have a slower metabolism, be insulin-resistant, or hypothyroidal. In that case, eating things like pizza or fried rice on a regular basis might swing much of the ratio of your weight gains toward fat. You are encouraged to eat until you're full all the time on this program, but if you start seeing two chins or suddenly becoming unable to fit into your jeans, it's time to clean up the fat in your diet. You don't need a lot of fat to meet your requirements, so keep that in mind as you eat your way up to your new body.

Bars And Shakes

As you probably know if you have ever picked up a bodybuilding magazine, a lot of weight trainers these days use bars and shakes to make eating at such frequent intervals more feasible. Most people don't have the luxury to sit down every two hours and eat a chicken breast, a potato, and some broccoli. But they can take a minute to eat a bar or drink a shake a couple more times during their workday. These tools can allow them to more easily fulfill their nutritional requirements, particularly for protein. Do you need bars and shakes? I believe the only time you absolutely need a shake is right after training. For all other meals, there is no advantage of bars and MRP's except convenience. If you could sit down every two hours to eat a solid meal, I think the only shake you would ever need would be the one after training. Food is the ultimate supplement, and your body is designed to process it perfectly. Bars are great because they are very portable and easily stored. You don't need to mix them, or keep them refrigerated. They can fit into a pocket, a fanny pack, a briefcase, or a gym bag. Bars are the perfect backup for those times when a meal is unavoidably postponed. Say you get to a restaurant, and you're already way past your limit for having eaten. Your stomach is rumbling. A quick look into the crowded lobby tells you that there is at least an hour wait just to get a table. You know you won't be seeing any food for at least 90 minutes. Why would you want to wait that long to eat and further impede your recovery process? If you carry a bar or two with you at times, as I do, you eat that sucker and alleviate the hunger pangs, not to mention catabolic condition, that you were experiencing. Shake packets are also pretty easy to carry around, although they do involve mixing up with water. In a perfect world where your training and eating were never interfered with, you wouldn't need to worry about portable meal 'backups,' but in this busy day and age we all can benefit from them at times to keep us on track nutritionally.

Other Supplements

There are many other products that you may find useful in your weight gaining plan. Creatine monohydrate has been proven to help in actual weight gain, primarily by attracting more water into the muscle cells, and also be enhancing your strength and endurance. Various other products may also be beneficial, though only creatine has a wealth of studies using human athletes as test subjects that prove conclusively its effectiveness. MCT oils can help you add calories and boost your energy for training. MCT's are a medium-chain triglyceride, a type of fat that the body treats like a carbohydrate. And, to increase your intensity in the gym, many trainers rely on caffeine and ephedrine products. Though these items are touted as fat burners, it is their stimulant effect that I feel is most useful. If you're worried about the long-term effects of these pills, you can get the same boost from a strong cup of coffee or espresso.

Structuring Meals

Now it's time to put all this information together. Here is a sample weight gain diet I did for one of my clients recently. The Parrillo supplements he uses could be substituted with those from any reputable company. This should give you a more cohesive idea about what a successful day of eating will look like.

Meal 1: 7:00 AM	Protein(g)	Carbs (g)	Fat (g)	Calories:
7 egg whites,	28	7	0	140
2 whole eggs (any style)	14	2	12	172
1 cup cooked oatmeal	6	25	2	142
1 scoop Hi-Protein Powder	15.5	4	0	160
1 Essential Vitamin tablet	--	--	--	--
1 Mineral Electrolyte tablet	--	--	--	--
Totals:	63.5	38	14	614

Meal 2: 9:30 AM	Protein(g)	Carbs (g)	Fat (g)	Calories
1.5 scoops Hi-Protein Powder	23.25	6	0	120
1.5 scoops Optimum Whey(mixed in water)	24.75	3	0	100
1 Essential Vitamin tablet	--	--	--	--
1 Mineral Electrolyte tablet	--	--	--	--
Totals:	48	9	0	220
Meal 3: 10:30 AM				
2Hi-Protein bars	40	60	6	460
1 Essential Vitamin tablet	--	--	--	--
1 Mineral Electrolyte tablet	--	--	--	--

Meal 4 12:00 PM	Protein(g)	Carbs (g)	Fat (g)	Calories
1.5 Chicken breasts	40.5	0	9	247.5
White Rice, 1.5 cups cooked	4.5	58.5	0	252
Broccoli, 1 cup	5	7	0	48
1 Essential Vitamin tablet	--	--	--	--
1 Mineral Electrolyte tablet	--	--	--	--
Totals:	50	65.5	9	547.5
Meal 5 2:30 PM				
1.5 scoops Hi-Protein Powder	23.25	6	0	120
1.5 scoops Optimum Whey(mixed in water)	24.75	3	0	100
1 Essential Vitamin tablet	--	--	--	--
1 Mineral Electrolyte tablet	--	--	--	--
Totals:	48	9	0	220

Meal 6 3:30 PM	Protein(g)	Carbs (g)	Fat (g)	Calories
2 Energy Bars	28	70	12	460
1 Essential Vitamin tablet	--	--	--	--
1 Mineral Electrolyte tablet	--	--	--	--
Cytomax 1 serving at 5:30 PM	– information not available –			
TRAIN 6 PM				
Meal 7 7:30 PM (Post–Workout shake)				
3scoops 50/50 Plus	30	25.5	0	225
2 cups nonfat (skim) milk	15	24	0	160
Totals:	45	49.5	0	385

Meal 8 8:30 PM	Protein(g)	Carbs (g)	Fat (g)	Calories
Tuna, 4 oz can in water	33	0	2	148
Baked Potato (medium size)	3	36	0	156
Carrots, 1 cup	2	11	0	52
10 Liver Amino tablets	15	0	0	0
1 Essential Vitamin tablet	--	--	--	--
1 Mineral Electrolyte tablet	--	--	--	--
Totals:	53	47	2	356
Daily Total:	375.5	348	43	3,262.5

For those of you who didn't think that many feedings could be squeezed into a day, now you see that they indeed can. This diet plan should also be able to show you how bars and shakes can be utilized by a person with a typical 9-5 office job to get all the proper nutrients in.

Getting Ripped

Something has definitely happened to our society over the past decade. Standards for how much or how little bodyfat you need to be considered lean have risen several degrees. Showing extreme muscular definition used to just be something competitive bodybuilders worried about, but now everyone and his cousin wants a clear, deep six-pack of abs, etched intercostals, and grooved obliques. Our movie stars like Brad Pitt and Gerard Butler are ripped in movies like *Fight Club* and *300*, and the male models in GQ and in Calvin Klein print ads and commercials look like they've been living on a Stairmaster and eating only carrot sticks for a year. Fat-burning pills and ab machines are a billion-dollar industry, as we are bombarded with lean bodies on TV shows, music videos, and magazine covers.

The Secret To Getting Ripped

All these companies want you to think that they have discovered the secret to getting ripped with little or no effort. The truth of the matter is that there is no secret except effort. Modifications in your diet and dedicated cardiovascular exercise on a regular basis are the only things that are going to make any significant impact on your bodyfat levels. Get the idea out of your head that some pill or exercise gadget is going to make it happen. Only you can make it happen. I will outline to you exactly the way to eat and do your cardio to melt away the ugly fat and reveal your true muscular physique below. I also want to make the point that these methods will work regardless of whether you are a man or a woman, a bodybuilder, workout enthusiast, or anything in between. None of it is really overly complicated, but the facts have been suppressed by those who wish to make a financial killing off the ignorance of the average person looking to lose weight.

Fad And Crash Diets

Fad diets and crash diets are all methods that will work in the short term. Most of them do so at the expense of losing an equal ratio of muscle and fat. Since 99% of dieters want the reward of seeing fast weight loss on the scale, these diets continue to lure people in with promises of dropping 20-30 pounds in a month. The Atkins Diet has you eating as much protein and fat as you like, but forbids carbohydrates. Since carbohydrates attract water, cutting them out of your diet will indeed cause you to lose several pounds almost immediately – several pounds of water, not fat. You do go on to lose fat, but after going without carbs for more than a couple months, cravings get the best of most folks. They break down and splurge on carbs. Only now their bodies are more insulin-sensitive than ever before, and they gain all the fat back and then some. Crash diets like "The Hollywood Diet" have you only drinking fruit juice, eating no solid food at all. With no dietary protein, your body will cannibalize its own muscle tissue for its essential amino acids. Is that the kind of weight loss you want? None of these fad diets can be followed forever. At some point you will go off the diet and gain back the fat, plus a little more. This is yo-yo dieting, a vicious circle that millions of overweight people are caught up in. Anything that extreme is doomed to fail.

Where Are You Starting From?

Before we get into the nuts and bolts of what you need to do, it's important to note that your results are going to take longer if you are carrying a great deal of extra bodyfat. Going from 20 % fat to 8 % is a lot easier than starting from 50 % or more. The plan is the same, the difference is in how long it will take to get down to single-digit bodyfat levels. For anyone to tell you their plan or product will get you shredded in thirty days or some random number is outrageous. It's realistic to lose one to two pounds a week of fat while preserving your lean muscle mass, or in some cases building more muscle. You may find it useful to have a body composition test performed by a certified personal trainer at your gym or health club. Most athletic departments at colleges and universities also offer this as a service either free of charge or for a small fee. This takes the guesswork out of knowing exactly where you are starting from. Most times someone will simply look in the mirror and estimate their rough bodyfat. The problem with this is that most people have little sense of accuracy. They may think they're somewhere around ten percent when it's over twenty. Nine times out of ten when people guess at their bodyfat percentage, they seriously underestimate. Have it done either with skin calipers, hydrostatic weighing, or bio-electric impedance. This will tell you how many pounds of fat you have, and how many pounds of lean tissue (muscle, bone, connective tissue). Now you will know exactly how many pounds of fat you must lose to get ripped. What constitutes being ripped, exactly? No one can put an exact number, as we all carry our bodyfat in slightly different ways, but for men you certainly have to get down to somewhere around 5-7 % to see all the details clearly in the midsection and elsewhere. Women look very lean at 10-12 %. Not everyone desires to achieve this level of condition, so adjust your goal accordingly. Men will still look very good, though not "ripped," at 10 %, women at about 15. If you discover you have forty pounds of fat to lose to get to the point you wish, count on taking a few months to reach it. I could prescribe a crash diet with excessive cardio to get you there much faster, but you would end up looking and feeling horrible, more like a concentration camp survivor than a fit, athletic person. My plan also emphasizes maximum retention of muscle mass. What good would it do you to get ripped if all your muscle is gone in the end? Slow, gradual fat loss is the right way to get lean and stay lean without any drastic, unhealthy measures. Now you're ready to learn about the diet.

Diet

Rather than think of this as a "diet," a more manageable term would be "changing the way you eat." Most of us associate the word 'diet' with suffering and deprivation, because that's what most people believe is the way to lose fat. My plan is quite the opposite. You're actually going to be eating plenty of nutritious food, probably more than ever before. In fact, the first subject I want to cover is meal frequency. The major change you will make is that you will be eating "clean" food that your digestive system will be able to process in less than three hours. Feeding your body this often is going to drastically speed up your metabolism, training it to operate at a higher level of efficiency. If you have been only eating the traditional three squares, you have instead been conditioning your metabolism to slow down to cope with the long spans of hours without eating. This is a survival mechanism built into all of us, left over from the caveman days when our ancestors often had to survive for many days without anything to eat. Here is the general rule about digestion to follow: a clean solid meal takes 2-3 hours to digest, depending on the individual. If you feel hungry at the two-hour mark, that's an indication that the food has passed from the stomach into the large intestine to begin the process of nutrient absorption and waste removal. Liquid meals like shakes will digest in 60-90 minutes, depending on thickness. Bars are about the same. Thus, it is realistic for you to consume 5-7 "meals" over the course of a day. It may sound crazy that eating this often will make you leaner, but hundreds of thousands, if not millions, of bodybuilders have proven this strategy works. The biggest mistake most overweight people make is not eating enough all day. By the time dinnertime comes, they are so ravenous that they devour everything that isn't moving. Then they go to sleep, slowing down their metabolisms and ensuring that most of the food they just ate is stored as fat. Don't fall into this very common trap. Don't be afraid to eat, because eating more often is going to play a huge role in losing the fat that you want to.

Now for the detailed stuff. What can I eat, and can't I eat? Obviously, the first thing you need to eliminate are useless, junk calories. Here's a short list:

What To Avoid

Candy, non-diet soda, white bread, rolls, pastries, donuts, cookies, thick sauces and dressings (try low-cal, fat-free dressings), cake, ice cream, pizza, butter, margarine, gravy, mayonnaise, fried foods, the vast majority of fast food, deli meats, and especially deep-fried foods. Also stay away from peanut butter, peanuts, hot dogs, french fries, granola bars (full of sugar), macaroni and cheese, potato or egg salad, olive and sunflower oils.

Next are foods that, although nutritious, make it difficult to lose bodyfat: dairy products such as milk, yogurt, and cheese (due to the milk sugar lactose), pasta (though whole-wheat pasta is okay), fruit juice (pure fructose, or fruit sugar), high-fat meats like pork, bacon, sausage, ham, lamb chops, and fatty cuts of red meat. Also be very wary of fruit smoothies and coffee concoctions. For instance, a "Coffee Coolata" from Dunkin' Donuts has over 400 calories – as much as a large order of French fries from McDonald's. But how many people drink these every day and simply assume they're just having a harmless cup of coffee with some flavor?

The core of your meals is always going to be lean protein sources like chicken breasts, turkey breasts, lean fish like tuna, cod, and orange roughy (salmon, trout, and mackerel are quite fatty), egg whites (a whole egg for every four to five whites is fine), and lean cuts of red meat like flank steak and ground sirloin. Avoid ground beef unless you can drain the fat out as you cook it, because even what is loosely called "97 % fat-free" ground beef is still in actuality nearly 40 % fat in its caloric content. Forget deli meats, too, as they are loaded with fat and preservatives. Fresh meat is the way to go. Grill or broil everything, though you can fry eggs with something like Pam with impunity. Definitely do not fry anything in cooking oil! Because your fat intake is so low, take two tablespoons of flaxseed oil a day to provide your body with essential fatty acids. Beware of anything that claims to be either 'fat-free' or 'sugar-free.' Usually when something is fat free, like the infamous Entenman's line of cakes and pastries, it is loaded with sugar. Sugar will make you just as fat as fat will. 'Sugar-free' products are safer, but many of them add a lot of fat for flavor and texture. Fat and sugar-free products have been gaining popularity, yet Americans are fatter than ever before. Too many overweight men and women think either label is a license to eat the whole box at a sitting, guilt-free. They may be free from guilt, but the empty calories are still being shoveled in and contributing to larger stores of bodyfat.

Reading Food Labels

You absolutely must become an educated food shopper. If not, you will be sabotaging your fat-loss efforts by buying fattier food than you think you are. Food labels are often deceptive, as they use every legal loophole the FDA and USDA allow to trick you. Ground meat is probably the best example. Fat percentages are determined by the weight of the fat in a given serving size. Surprisingly, fat is actually lighter than water. That's why grease floats on water. So when a package of ground beef is labeled as 90 % fat-free, take a look at the label. The first thing to look at is the amount of total calories per serving. Say it's 190 calories for an eight-ounce serving. Next, look at the 'calories from fat' or 'fat calories.' If it reads 70 or 80 calories, you can now see that this meat is far more than 10 % fat. 80 is far more than 10% of 190. It's actually more like 30-40 %. Ground turkey is equally problematic. You will see packages that are actually quite fatty are given names like "Extra Lean." Don't believe the name. The only ground turkey to safely buy is 100% ground breast. It's the most expensive kind, but that's because it's almost pure protein without all the worthless fat.

Food Values

The most complete resource for food values I have found so far is on a website that your tax dollars are paying for (if you're in America, that is.) It's: www.nal.usda.gov/fnic/cgi-bin/nut_search.pl

At this site, you can type in any kind of food, specify the serving size, and it will give you the most detailed breakdown you can imagine. It goes way beyond just calories, protein, and carbs, giving you the exact vitamin and mineral contents, lipid profiles, and even the quantity of each individual amino acid. There are also links on the home page that go into far greater detail about reading food labels than I did here.

Carbs: Yea Or Nay?

Carbs are a controversial subject lately due to the popularity of zero-carb diets like the Atkins Diet. The truth is that carbs in and of themselves do not make you fat. Eaten at the wrong times and in excess, and you bet they will turn to lard. Here's the easy way to have your carbs without guilt. Every day, have some carbs with breakfast to support normal brain function. Oatmeal, cream of wheat, or grits are the best choices because they are low-glycemic and take longest to digest. If breakfast happens to be the meal before you train with weights, you can eat a lot more without guilt. If you train later in the day, have some carbs with the last meal before you go to the gym. Good choices are potatoes, oatmeal, grits, brown rice, yams, and cream of wheat. After your workout, which may also include cardio, have a shake with 30-60 grams of whey protein and 40-80 grams of carbs in the form of maltodextrin (a medium chain carb found in any GNC or nutrition store as a carb powder). These ranges are on a scale proportionate to your lean bodyweight, or how much muscle you carry. A 150-pound man without a lot of muscle mass would be on the low end, and a 220-pound bodybuilder with a great deal of muscle would be at the high end. If you train in the morning or early afternoon, the next solid meal after this should include some carbs. If instead you train at night, the shake will be your last feeding with carbs. You can still have a lean protein serving and vegetables before going to bed, but no more carbs. Treated this way, carbs will be used as fuel for your weight training and also to refill the empty muscle glycogen reserves afterward. As for the amounts of carbs, you will have to fine-tune this yourself. If you do not see progress in bodyfat reduction, gradually reduce your carb totals. Do not be tempted to eliminate carbs completely, as they serve a very valuable function in your nutrition program. All of your other meals will be either a lean protein and vegetables (preferably raw), or a protein shake. Avoid "weight gainer" shakes which are loaded with sugar, and instead get a product that has ten grams or less of carbs per serving. You can find many varieties of powders which are either pure whey protein or a mix of whey and casein (milk protein), and both types have negligible amounts of carbs. If you eat bars, also be wary of their carb content. Many bars have as much sugar as regular candy bars. Always read your food labels carefully. One last thing. You may have heard that it's okay to have entire cheat days. Sorry, but doing that will slow down your fat loss by a huge margin. A moderate cheat meal once a week (a couple slices of pizza, not a whole pie, a cup of ice cream and not the whole quart) is fine, but a whole cheat day will easily drag what would normally take you ten weeks out to twenty weeks or more. Whenever you crave junk, just keep telling yourself that those ripped abs are going to feel better than the fleeting satisfaction of a donut or a pizza. Besides, haven't you already eaten enough crap in your life up to this point? It's time to start feeding your body clean fuel instead of garbage. Your body deserves it.

Sample Diet

Here's an example of the type of eating that will promote fat loss. The supplements listed are randomly chosen, and should not be considered an endorsement (and may not even be on the market by the time you read this). You can use any type of shakes and bars, as long as you carefully read the labels to be sure they are not loaded with sugar.

Meal 1: 7:00 AM	Protein(g)	Carbs (g)	Fat (g)	Calories:
7 egg whites,	28	7	0	140
2 whole eggs (any style)	14	2	12	172
1 cup cooked oatmeal	6	25	2	142
Multivitamin/ mineral Vitamin tablet	--	--	--	--
Totals:	48	34	14	454
Meal 2 10:00 AM				
Met-Rx Bar	32	15	8	290
Totals:	32	15	8	290
Meal 3 12:00 PM				
1.5 Chicken breasts	40.5	0	9	247.5
White Rice, 1.5 cups cooked	4.5	58.5	0	252
Broccoli, 1 cup	5	7	0	48
Multivitamin/ mineral Vitamin tablet	--	--	--	--
Totals:	50	65.5	9	547.5

Meal 4 3:30 PM	Protein(g)	Carbs (g)	Fat (g)	Calories:
Met-Rx Protein Plus Shake	46	15	0	210
Totals:	46	15	0	220
TRAIN – 6 PM				
Meal 5 7:30 PM				
Halibut, 8 oz	48	0	2	210
Baked Potato (medium size)	3	36	0	156
Carrots, 1 cup	2	11	0	52
Multivitamin/ mineral Vitamin tablet	--	--	--	--
Totals:	54	47	2	518
Daily Total:	230	176.5	33	2,029.5

This particular man trained relatively late in the day, which is why I included carbs at his final meal. If you train earlier in the day, you should have a shake containing whey protein and simple carbs like dextrose (table sugar) or maltodextrin immediately after training, then complex carbs with your next meal 60-90 minutes later.

Cardio

Your diet is handled, now let's get to the cardio. For your cardio to do its job and burn the fat away, you have to do it without any glycogen in your body. In other words, you must be in a carb-depleted state. Otherwise, your body will just use the glycogen to fuel the aerobic exercise and no bodyfat will be burned. The two best times to do your cardio are first thing in the morning on either an empty stomach or having only consumed protein, and immediately following your weight-training workout. Feel free to perform any type of cardio you like except swimming, which doesn't allow the body's core temperature to rise high enough. Another harsh reality is that your cardio must be intense. Walking at a leisurely pace on a treadmill simply doesn't burn enough calories for our purposes. What is far more effective is interval training, or working up to brief all-out "sprints" of effort, then slowing down just long enough to recover for the next interval. Gradually increase both the length and intensity until you are doing a total of 45-60 minutes a day, 4-6 days a week. A way to make it fun with most machines is to keep track of how many calories you burn in a session on the display, then trying to beat it by even just a calorie or two the next time. Get yourself an MP3 player with your favorite tunes that make you feel like moving, and work that fat off.

Supplements

Fat burners can give you an extra boost if you are doing everything else correctly with your diet and cardio. Do not count on them as miracle workers to take the place of a clean diet and adequate cardio. There are a number of fat-burners and thyroid stimulators on the market, most remarkably similar in formulas. Certainly you can take them for an added edge to speed up the process, but definitely do not rely on them or try to use them to make up for eating junk. I wrote an article in the *Musclemag International* Abdominals special issue in early 2000, most of which dealt with the right ways to eat and do cardio to shed fat. I mentioned fat-burners very briefly as being something that could be of some assistance. For almost two years I got e-mails about the article, and 99% of them were asking about how to use the fat-burners. Often they threw in a couple questions about cardio or nutrition that were already answered in the article. This tells me that they skimmed through the article until they saw something about a product that they believed would do the work for them. This never makes me very popular, but no supplement is ever going to take the place of hard work and discipline. Supplements can give you around 5-10 % faster results than not using them, so if you're in a hurry they could be useful for you.

How Weight Training Helps

Few people consider weight training to be important to the process of losing fat, and this is a mistake. Intense workouts with weights actually burn more calories per hour than all but the most rigorous cardio sessions. This also raises your metabolic rate and keeps it going for many hours after your workout is over. Cardio has this effect, but it doesn't last nearly as long. Another little-known fact is that muscle is very metabolically active. It demands a constant supply of energy from the body just to maintain itself. That means that a 200-pound muscular man burns far more calories just sitting down watching television than a 200-pound obese man does. This is also why men and women who carry an extreme amount of muscle tissue can get away with eating quite a bit more calories and even 'junk' than the average person, without getting fat. Even if you have zero desire to gain any muscle mass, you should still engage in at least three weekly sessions with weights to stimulate your metabolism and crank up the thermogenesis (fat burning). Unless you take in a surplus of calories and make a concerted effort to lift heavy, you will never have to worry about getting overly muscular. As many dedicated bodybuilding hopefuls can attest to, getting 'big muscles' isn't something that happens by accident. And if you shrug off weight training as being worthwhile only for those who are trying to get extremely big and strong, you are going to miss out on something that can increase your body's fat-burning by a huge percentage. Keep your reps in the range of 8-12 with as much resistance as you can safely handle for the upper body, and 15-20 reps for the lower body.

The Importance Of Patience

Before you begin this journey to a leaner you, it is critical that you understand that patience is a large part of your success. Despite crazy ad claims, fat loss is a fairly slow and gradual process. The first couple weeks are a bit deceptive, as this is when the rate of fat loss is actually quite rapid in many cases. Things do tend to slow down once the body gets over the initial shock of dealing with less calories, a cleaner diet, and the added cardiovascular activity. Because the process is so relatively slow, you won't be able to detect big changes from day to day in the mirror or on the scale. This has led to millions of people giving up on a proper nutrition program prematurely, when they certainly would have reached their goals in time. The rate that most of us are able to lose weight without sacrificing muscle mass is one to two pounds a week. Anything beyond that amount is almost surely going to consist of equal parts fat and muscle. A gradual weight loss is safer from a health perspective than a rapid loss, and is less likely to result in an episode of binge eating that puts most of the fat back on. Having your bodyfat tested is a very useful tool in setting your time frame for fat loss. If your goal is to lose twenty pounds of fat, you know that will take ten to twenty weeks. I know that sounds like far too long to most of you, but again I must stress the importance of maintaining your muscle mass. Anyone can cut their calories in half and do two hours of cardio a day to lose weight faster, but much of this will be from your lean muscle tissue. Doing it the way I recommend will keep you stronger, more energetic, and with far less suffering and hunger pangs than a crash diet will give you.

How Many Calories?

You may be wondering exactly how many calories a day you need to be consuming. Though many people in the fitness industry have attempted to prescribe cookie-cutter formulas to follow, none of them will be totally accurate. We all have different metabolic rates, activity levels, etc. The one thing that is certain is that you need to consume less calories than your body burns in a day, also called being in a state of caloric deficit. Rather than try to estimate this out of thin air or based on your height and weight, your best bet is to keep a food diary. In it you record everything you eat, listing the serving size and the amount of calories. Until you can start estimating serving sizes with a good degree of accuracy, a food scale to weigh your portions is needed. You can find these at www.parrillo.com or anywhere baking supplies and pans are sold. Gradually lower your calories by no more than 100 per week until you start to see the rate of fat loss you are satisfied with. Do NOT lower your calories all of a sudden. This is a guaranteed way to lose muscle as well as any energy you may have had. Once you find the caloric level that works best for you, don't go any lower than that. If anything, burn more calories in your cardio rather than starve yourself. Remember, when you're eating clean food, you can eat a much higher volume of food and the calorie count is still low in relation to the typical greasy American meal.

More On Cheat Meals

Any long-term nutrition program has to incorporate cheat meals, both for physiological and psychological reasons. For one thing, eating only clean food and lower calories for long periods will cause the body to downshift the metabolism eventually. Our bodies are excellent at adjusting to virtually anything. One way of confusing the metabolism is to occasionally eat a meal with far more calories and fat than what it has been accustomed to. So once a week, have your pizza or cheeseburgers. In this situation, far less of the junk will be converted to bodyfat stores. This is not, however, a free pass to eat everything in sight. It's only one meal a week, and even then you should avoid eating until you have to unbutton your pants. Try to save it for a time when you're going out to a restaurant or a special dinner you can look forward to. Some other sources may tell you it's okay to have a whole cheat day, but this will seriously undermine your fat-loss efforts and slow down your progress. You can eat a lot of crap over the course of a day and night, and don't think a food orgy like this isn't setting you back. One reasonable cheat meal a week is perfect. If you are seriously craving junk and going out of your mind, try drinking diet soda or eating low-calorie fruits like strawberries in moderation. If you can find snacks that are both fat-free and sugar-free, these are also an acceptable dessert in moderation.

Final Recommendations

One thing I highly recommend is that you take before and after pictures. These will serve as testimony to your willpower and dedication. As you lose more and more fat, you will become ever prouder of how far you have come from the before picture. Putting them somewhere like your refrigerator where you can see them constantly will reinforce your goals and confirm your achievements. Another trick is to buy a nice outfit that you can't yet fit into. Everyone wants to look great in nice clothes, so this will serve as further fuel to stick to your program. Also, you could do something like book a vacation a few months down the line somewhere where you know you'll be wearing a swimsuit. Having a deadline like this will give you a greater sense of urgency to lose the fat. If you have a friend or relative in a similar situation, perhaps you could make a little competition to see who can look better in three months time. Anything else you can think of to keep you focused is recommended, because the biggest obstacle to losing fat is inside each of our own heads.

A Word On Genetics

Before we finish, I do want to acknowledge that losing fat is indeed much harder for some people than it is others. If you legitimately have an underactive thyroid gland, then you should be on medication to regulate it. Glands aside, we all have different metabolisms. Some people can eat everything in sight and be thin as a rail, others can eat much less food and be obese. For some of you the process of fat loss will take a bit longer as a result, and that's just a fact we can't change. What you can change are your eating habits and your activity level, and these will in turn achieve the desired results if you persevere.

Putting It All Together

Now you are armed with the truth about what it will take to go from where you are now to where you want to be. I have deliberately made an effort to help you understand the realities of fat loss, because we are all subjected to a barrage or lies and misinformation on a daily basis.

Follow the guidelines I have outlined in this chapter, and you will soon begin to lose more fat than you probably believed you were capable of. Stay motivated, stay disciplined, stay on track and you will succeed.

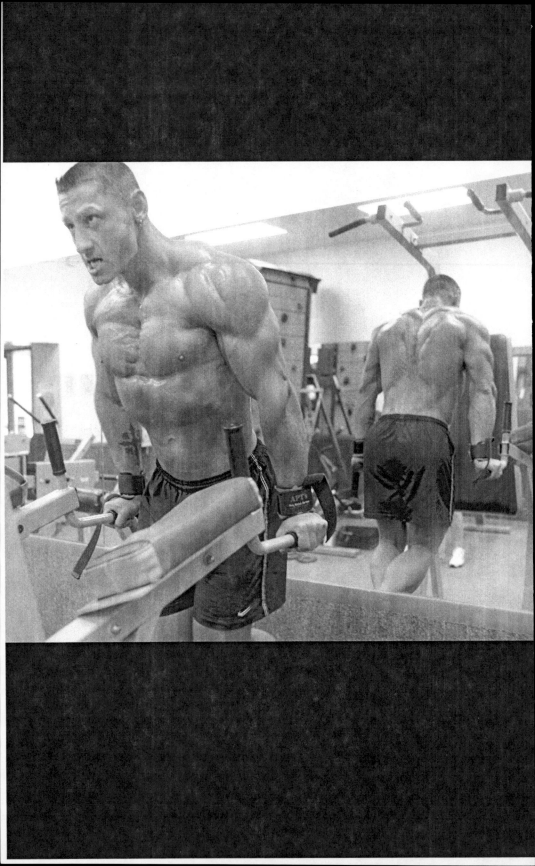

06

SUPPLEMENTS – SEPARATING FANTASY FROM REALITY

Do You Really Need Supplements?

Do you need supplements to get big and strong? The answer is, surprisingly, no. We know this to be true because men were getting big and strong for decades before supplements existed, simply by training hard with heavy weights and eating plenty of good food. And it's important to note that they usually only ate the standard three square meals a day back then, since it wasn't yet known how important it is to eat more frequently. So if you train hard and eat four or five solid meals every day, you will certainly have no trouble adding a substantial amount of muscle mass to your body.

However, there are many useful supplements, that, when added to that regimen, will improve your results by a wide margin. You can do without them, but you would do better with them.

The 10 Most Important Supplements for Bodybuilders

An In-the-trenches Perspective, Not A Sales Pitch

You probably know me as the guy who has been writing training articles for various other magazines for well over a decade. Occasionally I will touch on nutritional matters, such as when discussing how to eat for a six-pack or something along those lines. But by no means am I an expert on nutrition or supplements, meaning someone who can break everything down into molecular structure and chemical names to the last detail. There are no letters after my name because I don't have a degree in nutrition or chemistry. And I have no affiliation with any supplement companies, either. Wouldn't I seem an odd choice, then, to guide you through the ten most important supplements to invest your hard-earned dollars in? That's what I thought, too, but I do get asked about what types of supplements to use all the time, and I have formed my own opinions based on my experiences plus those of the many bodybuilders I know, all the way from rank beginners to top-three Mr. Olympia competitors. So here's what you won't be getting: a lot of highly technical scientific language, or products pushed on you because I have some financial interest in them (don't I wish!). You won't be getting a detailed explanation of what the products are and how they work – others are far better qualified than I to do that. You will be getting an honest assessment from someone who has been using supplements for close to twenty years, and whose advice on supplementation is sought out by many bodybuilders wanting to get the most benefit from the supplements they buy. I have no agenda other than a desire to help you in your quest to get the body you dream of.

Different Supplements For Different Goals

While some supplements fit into anyone's goals, there are others that are specifically geared toward adding muscle or losing fat. What I have taken into consideration in this list of the top ten 'must-have' supplements is effectiveness and necessity, or, what works, and what you really need. Usually, the marketplace is pretty good at weeding out products that don't deliver any results. Some of the clunkers over the years have included smilax, boron, HMB, myostatin blockers, and ecdysterones (bug steroids). If a product continues to sell well for a very long time, that's a reliable sign that enough people must be happy with it to keep it in production.

Forget Supplements If You Are Too Lazy To Eat Right

I learned over fifteen years ago from John Parrillo, a man who owns a supplement company called Parrillo Performance, that unless you are eating properly, you should not bother to spend a dime on supplements. It's true. So many bodybuilders, and even more folks who just work out for general health, fitness, and weight loss, look to supplements as magic potions that will do all the work for them. Unfortunately, it doesn't work that way. You need to fuel your body every two to three hours with protein, along with the right types of complex and fibrous carbohydrates and healthy fats. Top bodybuilders and fitness models look the way they do because they have dedicated themselves not only to hard and consistent training, but also consistent, clean eating. It's a lifestyle that never leaves meals to chance, and often they are cooked and packed ahead of time. When I explain the concept of eating five to seven moderate meals a day to most people, they think I'm out of my mind. "That's way too much work!" they protest, "I don't have time for that." Instead, they want to know what supplement they can buy to compensate for their missed meals, indulgences in junk food and alcohol, and generally poor diets. There is no such supplement, so if you're looking for it, good luck searching. Oh, don't worry, I am quite sure you will come across ads or infomercials promising that their product will give you the body of your dreams, but look for the fine print that says 'results not typical' or 'when combined with a proper exercise and nutrition program.' Now that I have gotten that out of the way, let's get rolling with the ten most important supplements as I see them.

1.   Protein Powders

I never hesitate to make this my first recommendation. Protein is the building block of muscle tissue, and you simply won't be able to make muscular gains without an adequate supply in your diet. How much bodybuilders actually need is a matter of debate, but the consensus always seems to fall somewhere between one to two grams per pound of bodyweight a day. Let's take the average there, a gram and a half, and apply it to a 170-pound lifter. This man would require 255 grams of protein per day. Now let's take a popular and cheap source of protein that many bodybuilders rely on – tuna fish. A can of chunk light has 33 grams of protein, which is also roughly what a chicken breast gives you. You would need almost nine of these a day to reach your requirement. Maybe you could do that for a day, or a few days, but even the most dedicated among us would eventually get sick of it to the point where just the smell of tuna would make them retch. Beyond that, chewing and swallowing all those solid meals is very time-consuming, and not everyone has the luxury of being able to drop what they're doing every two hours to sit down and eat a meal. Protein powders are a blessing in that they allow us to take in anywhere from a third to half of that total in the form of tasty shakes that can be drunk in just a minute. The term 'protein powders' covers a wide array of products, including whey protein, whey/casein blends, and MRP's (meal-replacement powders, the best-known brands being Mesotech by Muscletech, Met-Rx, and Myopex by EAS). All serve a unique purpose and should be used at different times. Whey digests very quickly and has minimal carbs, so it's best suited for those on a low-carb diet, or as a protein source before cardio, or as part of a post-workout shake (which we'll get to next). Whey/casein blends take longer to digest and are more suitable as meal replacements, especially before bedtime or even during the night. Soy protein is often cheaper than all of these, but I consider it an inferior source that bodybuilders should steer clear of. Protein derived from milk and egg sources will serve your needs far better.

2.   Post-workout Shakes

As valuable as post-workout shakes are, I am truly at a loss as to why they aren't used by every single person that trains. Hard and heavy weight training depletes our bodies of amino acids, glycogen (the form of carbohydrate stored in the liver and muscles), and creatine. Think of your muscles at this time as sponges that have been wrung dry. The brief period of time immediately following your workout is a precious window of opportunity to load everything back in and get a jumpstart on the recovery process. Sure, you could go out and eat a good meal like chicken and rice, and that's what a lot of people do. But a smarter tactic would be to immediately get all those substances into your body in a form that would digest as rapidly as possible. Then, in a half-hour to an hour, go ahead and have that solid meal. I have been carrying a cooler with me to the gym with my post-workout shake in it for years, and enduring all kinds of stupid remarks like, "Hey, is that your lunch in there?" Meanwhile, I have kept growing and improving while all the wise-asses still look the same. A post-workout shake should contain whey protein, simple sugars such as glucose or dextrose, and for good measure I always toss in five grams of creatine monohydrate and ten grams of L-Glutamine (an amino acid known for enhancing recovery and staving off overtraining). You can make your own shake by getting the ingredients separately, or buy any of the products specifically designed for this purpose, such as Surge from Biotest, a combination of Muscletech's Cell-tech and Nitro-Tech like Jay Cutler uses, or Recover-X from Muscle-Link. Again, I have to say that these are not product endorsements, just examples of popular brands. By the time you read this, there will be several more on the market, as post-workout nutrition has been gaining more momentum as something understood to drastically enhance recovery.

3.   Multi-vitamin/mineral And Antioxidants

I know, this one doesn't sound too exciting or exotic, does it? Maybe not, but trust me when I say that this is one type of product that you should all be taking, every day, even if it doesn't have any cool before-and-after ads or promises to add fifty pounds to your bench press.

The foods we eat these days have been so processed that many of the important vitamins and minerals have been leeched out of them. And our environment, from the air we breathe, to the water we drink and bathe in, and any other number of chemicals we come in contact with every day in everything from shampoo to exhaust fumes, is chock full of toxins and carcinogens. Taking a multivitamin/mineral along with antioxidants every day is a very inexpensive way to cover your bases and protect yourself from this barrage of threats. There are any number of multivitamin/mineral products out there such as Centrum, and in the same section of your grocery store or GNC you will see the antioxidants. Look for those that contain vitamin E, beta-carotene, vitamins B2, B3, and B6, CoEnzyme Q-10, bilberry, pine bark, grape seed, selenium, zinc, gingko biloba, and copper. There is also substantial evidence to support taking additional vitamin C every day. These aren't the most glamorous products out there, but they will contribute to your overall health, and that can only be a positive factor toward improving your physique.

4. Creatine

Very few products have stood the test of time the way creatine has. First introduced to bodybuilders in the early 1990's, creatine has since been proven both effective and safe in hundreds of university studies. It increases muscular strength and endurance, as well as hydrates the muscle cells, or attracts more water into them. This causes a weight gain, and even though it's only water, it's very satisfying for someone who has been stuck at the same weight for months or years to suddenly get on the scale and see five to ten pounds more. And since you can train with a little more weight and get a few more reps, as creatine helps fuel muscular contractions at the molecular level, you will also build more actual muscle mass. Basically, you can't go wrong with creatine, which is why it is still an incredibly popular product used by millions of bodybuilders, regular gym members, and athletes in every sport all the way from high school to the pro's and the Olympics. There are many versions out these days, so you have your choice. To be on the safe side, stick with products from known companies like Muscletech, Twinlab, Pinnacle, Optimim Nutrition, and others. There have also been many 'advanced' types of creatine introduced, such as micronized creatine, creatine ethyl ester, creatine malate, and more. While they all promise to be more effective than the basic creatine monohydrate, keep in mind that all the studies done in the critical first decade of its use showing it was safe and effective as a supplement used the monohydrate form – which is also the least expensive by far of all the types you can buy.

5.   L-Glutamine

L-Glutamine is an amino acid used by bodybuilders hoping to enhance their recovery and avoid overtraining. There is not a whole lot of actual research to back this up, but there is enough anecdotal evidence from the many thousands that have used it and testify to its effectiveness to justify using it. It does appear to be more valuable for those with heavy and frequent training volumes who are at a high risk of overtraining. So if you only train three times a week, you may not really benefit from L-Glutamine. But if you train five or more times a week, or if you have a physically demanding job, it's probably a good idea to invest in it. Most bodybuilders will take ten grams before training, ten grams after, and optionally, another ten grams right before bedtime.

6.   Joint Complex

Young guys getting into bodybuilding or just heavy weight training typically aren't too concerned with their joints. Why would they worry about something like that? I know that I thought I was indestructible as a teenager. We all did. Talk to guys in their thirties and forties, however, and they will let you know just how fragile and vulnerable the body truly is. A couple decades of heavy training can and often does lead to chronic pain in the elbows, knees, shoulders, lower back, and wrists. Not only is the pain annoying, but it often limits your training, even making certain exercises impossible to do anymore, and forcing you to go a lot lighter than you once did with others. I know you youngsters out there are glossing right past this, thinking 'it will never happen to me,' but you have to believe that it can and probably will. Aside from using good form and not going extremely heavy all the time, you can spare yourself future pain by taking a joint health complex. Regular use will help you strengthen and rebuild connective tissue, reduce inflammation and pain, increase joint flexibility, and speed the healing process of joint and connective tissue injuries, which is notoriously slow. You can find these anywhere from GNC, to Walgreens, or even Costco. Look for formulas that contain glucosamine sulfate, chondroitin, shark cartilage, SAMe, and MSM.

7.   Protein Bars

A major nutritional sin that keeps many from achieving their physique goals, whether those goals involve muscle gain, fat loss, or both, is missing meals. You absolutely must provide a steady stream of nutrients, particularly protein, to your body if you want to recover and grow from workouts, or to keep the metabolism running at an optimal rate to burn bodyfat. But it isn't practical or convenient for everyone to eat every two to three hours. Sometimes you may be driving, or running around, or at work and unable to even get to a shake stored in the refrigerator. Protein bars can be nutritional saviors by simple virtue of their portability. You can keep them in your pocket, your fanny pack, backpack, briefcase, in your desk at work, in the glove compartment of your car, etc. They travel well and they don't make a mess, as anyone who has ever spilled a shake all over their car or desk will appreciate. By keeping them around at all times, you have an emergency protein supply at your disposal to make sure you never miss out on this key macronutrient. The term 'protein bar' is pretty vague, as there are many types of supplement bars, with differing ratios of protein, carbs, and fat. Some have more or less sugar than others, as well as total caloric content. Choose the type that suits your needs. For instance, if you are trying to lose fat, you don't want a bar with a heavy load of sugar and calories, or even a lot of carbs. But if you're a hardgainer who needs plenty of calories and carbs, that type of bar would be ideal.

8.   Fat Burners

As I point out over and over again at the risk of getting on your nerves, losing bodyfat is mainly a factor of a clean diet and the right amount of cardiovascular exercise. With those things in place, a fat-burning product can speed up or enhance your results further. There are a huge variety of these products available. For a few years, the main ingredients in most were caffeine and ephedra. Now that the FDA has banned ephedra, it's a veritable chemistry lab out there. Some of the items you'll see in today's fat-burners include green tea, bitter orange, fenugreek, synephrine, yohimbe, guggulsterones, garcinia camboga, and good old caffeine, which never lets you down. You can find some that have stimulant properties as well as others that promise to be stimulant-free. That's important, because some people react very badly to stimulants, getting jittery, nervous, and have difficulty sleeping.

9. Tribulus Terrestris

Derived from a plant, tribulus helps to stimulate the body to produce more testosterone by leading to the production of luteinizing hormone (LH). As you should know, testosterone is the hormone that allows us to build muscle mass. Popular brands include Tribex from Biotest and Vitrix from Nutrex. I should add that those of you twenty-five years of age and under should already be producing plenty of testosterone on your own, and the use of tribulus or any other product designed to increase test production would be a waste of money. Lifters over the age of thirty to thirty-five will see far more benefits than younger men will. I should note that there are many 'hormonal' types of products available and many will deliver a noticeable anabolic effect. Two I have used successfully are Halodrol liquigels and Novedex XT from Gaspari Nutrition. There are literally hundreds more on the market. The same rules apply with respect to age, meaning younger guys will not get nearly as much out of these products as men over 35.

10. Essential Fatty Acids Or Fish Oil

We all know that protein plays a vital role in the process of muscle repair and growth, but how many are aware that an adequate amount of dietary fat is also necessary? Believe it or not, a lot of bodybuilders fail to get the results they want because they don't get enough fat in their diets. This is one area that the old-time bodybuilders actually were smarter about than today's lifters, despite the advantages of modern nutritional information and high-tech supplements. Some of their favorite muscle-building foods included red meat, whole milk, whole eggs, and nuts. And you know what? Considering that these guys were all drug-free until the early 1960's, they were pretty damned big and thick! Check out old pictures of John Grimek, Reg Park, Clancy Ross, Dan Lurie, George Eiferman, and Chuck Sipes. I assure you, that if these guys had been on steroids and other supplements, they would have been every bit as impressive as Ronnie, Arnold, or Dorian. Modern bodybuilders and weight trainers often completely avoid dietary fat, or at least don't get enough of it. They subsist on fat-free items like chicken breasts, egg whites, plain sweet potatoes, and plain oatmeal (with some Splenda). If that sounds anything like your meal plan, it's time you added in some healthy fats in supplement form. You have your choice of flax seed oil, Omega-3 fatty acids from fish, evening primrose oil, or CLA, all available in gel form. I have actually heard back from guys whose only change in training, diet, or supplements was adding some sort of EFA supplement in, and saw results within a couple weeks. I know it sounds crazy, but I swear it's true.

Those are ten supplements I feel totally confident that bodybuilders can't go wrong with. If you can afford to use all ten, I guarantee you they will make a difference in the way your physique looks and performs. With those, a spot-on eating plan, and intense training with adequate rest, you can expect to be at your physical peak – and that peak is a hell of a nice place to be!

Advertising Tactics – Buyer Beware

Advertising, by its very nature, is a business of influencing you to buy things you don't really need, or at least to buy the things you need from one company above all others. The tactics are powerful, using psychology, visual and audio stimulation, and playing to our deepest fears and desires.

The supplement industry is ruthlessly competitive and notoriously difficult to turn a profit in. After all, there are many products that seem remarkably similar to each other. Why are you going to buy Company

X's creatine instead of Company Y's? There are a few very common ways the ads will try to convince you that their product trumps all others, beyond the usual clever insinuations that using their brand will get you laid by the women of your dreams.

Tactic # 1 – Studies

Very often you will see statistics and numbers from a study that showed a product to be superior to others of its type, or that study subjects gained an average of twenty pounds of muscle or lost thirty pounds of fat using the product. Occasionally, these numbers reflect the truth, or at least the truth of the study. First of all, the only way you can find out how the study was actually conducted is if it was summarized in a peer-reviewed medical or trade journal such as *Journal of the American Medical Association* or *Journal of Sports Medicine Physical Fitness.* These will provide details that might make you think twice about the efficacy of the product, should you bother to find and read them. Most studies are conducted at universities and use students as test subjects. Often the students have little or no experience with serious weight training. Therefore, it really doesn't matter what supplements they use or don't use during the trial period. Because they are relatively new to training, they will make gains. Other studies with fat-loss have subjects that haven't been eating well or doing cardio. Other studies are done using very sick people. Some supplement may increase their testosterone levels or decrease their levels of catabolic hormones like cortisol. But to compare these types of test subjects to your average bodybuilder, who is strong, healthy, and has been training hard for years, is not very reliable. Even when athletes are used in studies, they are rarely bodybuilders – more often bicyclists or some other type of endurance athlete. This is not to say that all the studies and their results are pure chicanery, only that they don't always correlate to the results you would probably experience.

Tactic # 2 – Athlete Endorsements

I don't begrudge anyone from making a living, and bodybuilding is one of the least financially rewarding professional sports in existence. In the huge sports like football, baseball, and basketball, the star athletes are paid millions of dollars to endorse sneakers, soft drinks, sports beverages, and assorted items like wireless providers and snacks. In bodybuilding, the athletes are pretty much limited to supplements. And unfortunately, the contracts are a far cry from what their peers in other sports receive. As of this writing, Ronnie Coleman's 500-thousand-dollar deal with BSN in 2005 represents the largest of such contract. A handful of other top men are paid lower six-figure amounts. The vast majority of the pro's and top amateurs you see in ads are paid no more than thirty to sixty thousand dollars a year, and many more receive only free product as payment.

Still, the ads are a strain on credulity, since they typically take the tone of the athlete giving credit to the particular product for their development. Michael Jordan never claimed that Air Jordans made him the phenomenal athlete he was, yet such claims are rampant in bodybuilding magazines. To the seasoned consumer, such tactics fall flat on their face. For instance, if it's a new product and this bodybuilder has been a champion for many years, obviously a link can't be drawn between the product and his success, since the product didn't exist for most of his career. Another questionable issue is that very often, top athletes switch companies several times over the course of their careers. Either the company doesn't feel they are marketable any longer and drops them, or another company comes along and offers a lot more money. This makes it tough to believe an athlete truly believes in Company A, if in the past he has said the same things about companies B, C, and D. However, the target market for supplements isn't seasoned, mature bodybuilders. They are trying to convince the young guys aged 18-25 to part with some of their paycheck in hopes of looking like Mr. Olympia or Mr. USA. This market is far more impressionable and far more likely to idolize the freaky physique champions, since they haven't yet figured out that it's a combination of rare genetics, years of hard training and good nutrition, and of course, significant amounts of steroids and other drugs that make these men look so inhumanly buffed.

Tactic # 3 – Before And After Photos

Again, I feel the need to point out that the bodybuilding industry is far from unique in its use of before and after photos. Mainstream companies like Metabolife and Trimspa have utilized this type of ad to rake in untold millions of dollars, and at least one of them has been sued for false advertising. Before and after photos are especially compelling and convincing because they appear to show concrete proof that the product in question indeed delivers the promised results. These photos can be manipulated in any number of ways so that the after is dramatically different from the before. The most obvious method is airbrushing and other tricks of computer programs like Photoshop. But more often, no computer work on the photos is even needed. The subject is made to look as horrible as possible in the before photo. They have no tan, their hair is messed up, they look sad, and their posture is slumped and listless. If they are a woman, they have no makeup on. Often a man wears rumpled, loose shorts in the first photo and has excessive body hair. In the after photo, both the physique and the person's grooming are much improved. They are tanned, shaved, smiling, hair perfectly coiffed, and the body has changed in whatever way it was supposed to. In the fine print, you will see statements such as 'results not typical' and an asterisk above touting the results leads to small type informing you that the results were obtained 'in conjunction with a proper training and diet regimen.'

Many times, the before photo is taken of a bodybuilding, fitness, or Figure competitor just before they start their diet for a competition. This is the worst they usually look. Over the next six, eight, ten, or twelve weeks, whatever length of time passage the photos represent, the subjects eat better, do more cardio, tan, and often also use drugs that build muscle and reduce bodyfat. The after photos portray a dramatic transformation, but one that's nothing unheard of for those that know about contest preparation. Did the subjects use the products in question? Maybe, and maybe not. I distinctly remember one bodybuilder in the mid-1990's telling me how he sent the same sets of photos to ten different companies, hoping to get an endorsement, even going so far as to hold all their products in the photos! If that isn't bad enough, I have also heard of the 'time-reversal' trick. For that, the athlete takes the 'after' picture when he's in great shape, then stops training, eats like a pig, and takes the 'before' photo once he or she is sufficiently out of shape. There was one very famous ad that EAS came out with a decade ago that was allegedly this process in stages, starting with the model fat, and ending with him in great condition.

All this was not meant to discourage you from buying supplements. There are many effective products out there, as discussed earlier. It's just that the companies have no choice but to employ advertising tactics that could be interpreted as misleading in an effort to sway you to their company's products. Personally, I believe that all the major supplement companies are fairly equal in terms of quality and meeting label claims, so it comes down to personal preference and trial and error to see which brand you buy.

Can Supplements Make Up For Wimpy Training?

Earlier we discussed how supplements can not take the place of good nutrition. The other point that needs to be hammered home is that supplements can't replace hard training, either. There are supplements that can help you train harder, such as stimulants. But too often, lifters think of supplements as magic pills and potions that will turn them into huge, ripped gods of muscle. Unless you are putting in a lot of hard work with heavy weights in the gym, the only miracle you will experience is the disappearance of your money with nothing to show for it. I used to get quite disgusted with a kid named Pete at my old gym in Pasadena that was forever inquiring about the latest supplements whose ads he had been enthralled with. I was so annoyed because he trained with very little intensity, using weights that would hardly challenge a kitten. He, like so many others, did not understand the value of hard work in the gym. Instead, Pete and all the others like him out there put far too much importance on the role of supplements, and far too little emphasis on the actual training. Supplements work, in the sense that they can enhance your results if you are training properly and supporting that training with good nutrition and ample rest. If not, they are nothing more than a waste of money.

Postscript: A Changing Market

Due to the nature of the supplement industry, there will always be at least a couple new types of products introduced each year. As I write this in 2008, nitric oxide products like NO Xplode are extremely popular, for example. Typically, effective products stand the test of time and remain on the market, while those that bodybuilders don't feel are particularly effective (HMB, for example) quietly go away. Stay informed and try to buy only products that have both some science behind them as well as a track record among satisfied consumers. The message boards of site like www.GetBig.com, www.bodybuilding.com, www.musculardevelopment.com, and www.musclemayhem.com. All have sections where site members can post unbiased reviews. These are definitely worth checking out before you spend your hard-earned money on a product you're not sure about.

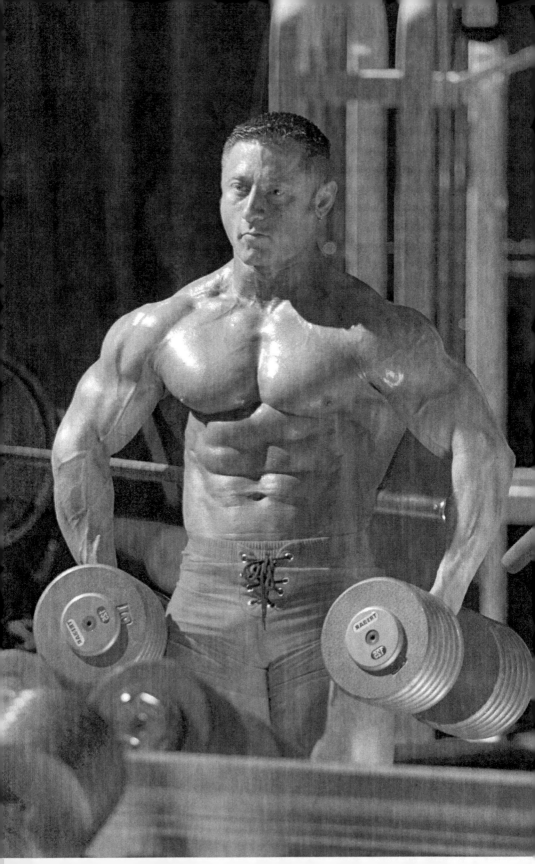

07

SECRETS OF THE CHAMPIONS

Do The Pro's Really Have Any Secrets?

One of the great pretenses of the bodybuilding industry, particularly of the magazines that I have made my living writing for full-time since 2000, is that pro bodybuilders are experts on the subjects of training and nutrition. Further, it's often either insinuated or blatantly claimed that these muscular marvels are privy to secrets that the average trainer has no inkling of. Having known, spoken to, and observed hundreds of pro's over the last seventeen years of my life, I can assure you that there are no such secrets. Pro bodybuilders train just like the vast majority of amateur bodybuilders. Neither their workouts nor nutritional programs differ too drastically from that of any good competitive bodybuilder from the regional level on up. There are no 'secret' bodypart routines that give them the awesome development they display. I will never forget one time in 1991 talking to Shawn Ray at the Gold's Gym in Fullerton, California, when he recounted an exchange between him and another gym member. The guy was desperate to have huge arms like Shawn, and begged to know what exercises he did for them.

"The same exercises as you, bro," he deadpanned. The young man's face fell, as this was clearly not what he was hoping or expecting to hear. As we discussed in an earlier chapter, genetics play an enormous role in the development of a person's muscles. That being said, the pro's tend to do a lot of things right. None of these things are secret or groundbreaking, but it always surprises me how few bodybuilders create the optimal environment for growth.

Just about every pro trains savagely hard. They train like it's their job, because it is. The contests are just a means to showcase the hard work in the gym that these men have been doing for years. Most pro's are very strong on a wide variety of free weight basics, like squats, bench presses, military presses, barbell rows, and so on. Some of them rely more on a mix of free weights and machines as they age, both because they have already built all the mass they need, or because nagging injuries make some free weight exercises too painful to perform anymore. But whether the pro's train heavy or not so heavy, with low or high reps, or how they split their bodyparts up throughout the week, they generally have found a training style that works for them, and they stick to it. They have also more or less settled on the exercises that they respond to best. Contrast this with the fickle average bodybuilder, who is forever searching for something new, and always convinced that nothing works very well for them. Pro's usually have more time on their hands to train than the average guy, but again this is due to the fact that they are professional athletes. They can go to the gym twice a day and do cardio two more times if they so desire. Often they don't have children or any other responsibilities to get in the way of their scheduled workouts and cardio sessions.

When it comes to eating, again the pro's treat it like a job, which is the only approach that guarantees full nutritional support for heavy training, as well as recovery from that training. Men like Jay Cutler and Victor Martinez eat around the clock, usually every two to three hours. They absolutely do not miss meals. If they are going anywhere where they won't be absolutely sure that the types of food they require will be available when they need it, they pack their own food and bring it along in a cooler. Gustavo Badell even did this when he took his wife and kids to Disneyland and Universal Studios, and when he was in the hospital as his wife was having their third child just before the 2007 Mr. Olympia. The very best bodybuilders are always conscious of when they need to eat, and plan to have all those meals ready and available at the appropriate times. Six-time Mr. Olympia winner Dorian Yates used to set the alarm on his wristwatch to go off right before mealtimes so he wouldn't forget. This should be a clear indicator that he didn't rely on his appetite to tell him when to eat. That's what most weight trainers do. Not only that, they usually don't have a clear idea of what they will be eating over the course of a day, when they will eat it, and where they will be at these times. Top bodybuilders never make any types of plans without considering how they will get their scheduled meals in first. To the average guy, that probably sounds like a pain in the ass, but it's this diligent attention to a constant supply of nutrients that is in large part responsible for the physiques of the pro's. Yes, they train hard, and sure, most use steroids (more on that soon), but without the right foods in the right amounts, at the right times, they would never look the way they do.

Pro's are also very conscious of minimizing stress and getting enough sleep. Stress is catabolic, and makes it harder to either gain muscle or lose fat. So pro's try not to deal with people or situations that cause them mental stress. When a contest is approaching, it's often difficult to get them on the phone because they may not be taking calls except from immediate family and friends. They will also turn off their phones when it's time to sleep, so they won't be disturbed. Many pro's take regular afternoon naps to further ensure adequate rest. Granted, the average person does not have the time to do this, but it does point out how the pro's set their lives up around training, eating, and sleeping to the best of their abilities, knowing that getting all three factors right is the real 'secret' that most people that lift weights don't seem to grasp.

Are Pro Bodybuilders Role Models?

NBA star Charles Barkley said it best when he uttered the famous declaration, "I am not a role model." Yet despite his honesty and attempt to discourage America from idolizing star athletes, we continue to glorify these talented men as being above human frailties. I am here to tell you that pro bodybuilders are indeed human, just like you and me. They are subject to all the same temptations, vices, and errors in judgment that anybody else is.

Recreational drug use is common, though by no means are the majority of pro bodybuilders addicts or even regular users. The percentage of rec drug users is higher than that of the general population, but that's probably due to the extreme and addictive type of personality that often gravitates to bodybuilding in the first place. Many men and women take up bodybuilding to fill some need or void, some loneliness, lack of attention, or insecurity. Despite my lack of psychological education, even I can recognize that these same feelings can and often do lead to taking solace in drugs that alter consciousness and numb pain, both physical and emotional.

For a time in the 1990's, a synthetic opiate called Nubain was spreading like a plague among the bodybuilding community. Stories abounded of various bodybuilders who were sliding deeper into addiction of the injectable drug. As the millennium passed, Nubain's popularity waned. Now it's mainly marijuana, cocaine, and 'club drugs' such as Ecstasy, Special K, and GHB that are rampant among the 'partying' segment of bodybuilders. All of these are preferable to alcohol, since they lack the empty calories and liver stress of booze (important, since steroids already tax the liver). Still, very few top bodybuilders use these drugs on a regular basis, with the possible exception of marijuana, which is used by some in the off-season to boost the appetite and relax. For the most part, top bodybuilders and fitness women save their recreational drug indulgences for after competitions, which they may or may not have competed in. These after-parties can reach heights of bacchanalia that would shock most of their fans, though it's nothing that doesn't happen in nightclubs all over the world every day. I have been to many of these after-parties, and in fact took some heat for recounting the goings-on. Not long before Craig Titus and Kelly Ryan concluded their downward spiral of drug use and questionable morality, Craig was very upset at my reports on their parties. Yet never have I claimed to be an angel myself. After all, how could I accurately write about these events without being part of them?

Since I have been accused of attempting to smear the sport of professional bodybuilding by portraying it as a gang of muscular degenerates, I would like to take this chance to set the record straight. There are many bodybuilders, all the way from non-competitors to Olympia finalists, that live very 'clean' and exemplary lives. They may use steroids to build their muscles, but they would never consider taking drugs just to get high. I have spoken to some men that have never so much as had a drink of alcohol or smoked a single cigarette in their lives, much less used recreational drugs. Many are deeply religious, and devoted to being good spouses and parents.

Next, what about the sex lives of top bodybuilders? Are they a bunch of promiscuous deviants, into orgies, partner-swapping, and prostitution? As with drug abusers, that element does exist in the sport, just as that subculture exists anywhere you go. An infamous account of one such group of bodybuilders on the West Coast called "The Sex Cult of Venice Beach" appeared online on a site called www.testosterone.net, and immediately caused an uproar. Some denounced it as exploitative fiction, while others claimed to know that such 'parties' did take place regularly. As for being promiscuous, I doubt that pro bodybuilders are any more so than athletes in other sports. The fact that they have such incredible bodies and a little bit of money and fame (albeit in a cult sport) does tend to make it easier for them to find willing partners. Rumors abound that many bodybuilders are bisexual. I can't either confirm or deny this, though I have heard plenty of stories. I have also heard that it's quite common for bodybuilders, and more often, female fitness and Figure competitors, to exchange sex for money, publicity, endorsement contracts, or other favors. But this type of thing exists in all types of business. The Hollywood 'casting couch' and the phrase 'sleeping his/her way to the top' are evidence of this. With the bodybuilding and fitness industry being so tough to make a decent living at, it's understandable that some would choose to sell their bodies in order to pay for expenses such as food, drugs, rent, and payments on luxury vehicles.

One thing that should be said is that steroids dramatically increase the sex drive. Since just about all top bodybuilders use steroids for at least half the year, it stands to reason that they will more actively seek out sex and sex partners than the average person might. This situation could, in theory, be responsible for more partners among single bodybuilders, and frequent infidelity among those that are married. But there are plenty of steroid-using bodybuilders that manage to keep their lust reigned in, and stay faithful to spouses or significant others.

Just How Much Juice Are These Guys On?

There is no doubt that pro bodybuilders today use far more steroids and other drugs than ever, both in terms of sheer quantity and variety. Back in the late 1960's and early 1970's, the days of Arnold, Sergio, and Dave Draper, the typical steroid 'stack' consisted of a few tabs of Dianabol and Winstrol each, and usually these were only used in the eight or ten weeks before a major competition – which were few and far between in that era. The scene has changed drastically since then. Now it's common for men to use a combination of three to five different steroids at once, plus growth hormone, insulin, IGF-1, anti-estrogens like Arimidex or Proviron, thyroid and asthma medications to lose fat, and at contest time, pharmaceutical diuretics to shed water from under the skin and heighten muscular definition. Weekly steroid totals can reach anywhere from 1,500 milligrams on the low end to five or six thousand on the high end. The base of many stacks is one to two grams (2,000 milligrams) of some form of injectable testosterone. And the scariest thing is that drug use is either year-round, or very close to it. Pro's today use steroids to build mass in the off-season and to maintain the freaky look for guest posing and other types of appearances. God forbid they show up anywhere without looking as huge as usual – jeering threads will pop up instantly on two dozen message boards laughing at how small they are. And since the IFBB contest schedule has events from February until October every year, those who compete in both the spring and fall shows are on steroids most of the time. They would prefer not to be in most cases, but they have no choice if they want to try and make a living at this sport. They know that most pro careers are realistically only five to ten years long, so they need to do as well as they can in that span of time before it's time to move on.

As for cash amounts that the pro's spend on their drug cycles, this has been the subject of debate and fodder for plenty of sensationalized articles with anonymous athletes. The fans seem fascinated with it, and love to hear ludicrous sums being discussed. You will hear figures ranging anywhere from fifty to a hundred thousand dollars a year being spent. Steroids themselves aren't all that expensive, until you start talking about the harder-to-find items generally used near contest time, like Masteron, Halotestin, Primobolan, and Anavar. It should be noted that as the federal government has made a point to crack down on steroids over recent years, prices have gone up across the board and availability has also been affected (hence the price gouging). Growth hormone is quite pricey. It's also true that since 9/11 has made it far more difficult to import steroids into the USA, prices have gone way up. All told, a pro bodybuilder might spend anywhere from ten to fifty thousand dollars a year on drugs. Average bodybuilders love to hear the highest estimates, because this becomes both a justification for why they don't look like the pro's (don't want to spend that much money) and an excuse (can't afford it). What's ironic is that there are plenty of amateur bodybuilders, and this even encompasses many that don't compete, who use just as much gear as the guys in the magazines. Yet because they lack the right genetics, don't train and eat right, or both, they look nothing like the pro's and top amateurs.

One misconception is that all the pro's are reckless in their drug use, and care less about their health and longevity than they do winning a contest or securing a big endorsement contract. There are a few out there with this kamikaze attitude, but most of the top bodybuilders I have ever known only use steroids because they feel they have no choice. If they don't use steroids, they will be beaten badly by those that do, or passed over for contracts by the freakier guys. In the past couple years, America has come to understand that this situation of athletes using drugs to stay competitive is by no means confined to bodybuilding. We now know that steroids are widely used even in respected arenas such as the Olympics and major league baseball. Unfortunately for bodybuilders, their extreme development makes their drug use far more obvious to the observer. After all, it is possible to hit a home run without steroids, but a man doesn't weigh 280 pounds at two percent bodyfat without them. But as I have tried to impress upon you several times, steroids do not turn just anyone into a pro bodybuilder. Only a lucky few have the requisite genetics, and even then, years of dedicated training and eating must be undertaken to build a pro-caliber physique. This fact will never be accepted by most, as it isn't as comforting as thinking that the pro's are all drug monsters that use quantities of steroids capable of blowing out the liver of a blue whale.

Lessons To Be Learned From The Pro's

We have established that without rare, gifted genetics and steady, long-term usage of a wide variety of drugs, nobody is going to look like the pro bodybuilders on the covers of the magazines. You could all too easily then dismiss them all as being of no use to the regular guy except in terms of motivation and inspiration. But there are a few things the pro's do that can and should serve to aid you in your own quest to build the best physique you are capable of.

The most important lesson you can take from these larger-than-life figures is *consistency*. They train hard and eat a lot of good food, not just once in a while, but all the time. Your own results will probably never be as fast or dramatic as theirs, but keep in mind that every tiny gain builds on the next and adds up to larger gains over time. I am living proof of this, as are many others that have been training for many years. Skipping workouts and meals, or even eating the wrong things too often, will only keep you further from reaching your goals.

Another trait you can take from the pro's is their *intense motivation to succeed*. If you ever speak to an elite bodybuilder, you can immediately sense that failure is not an option for them. They have a tremendous drive to be the best, which is often a carryover from younger years in other competitive sports. This fuels their workouts and provides the discipline to adhere to strict contest diets for anywhere from twelve to twenty weeks to reach contest condition. Doubt and apathy have no place in this regimen. They want to win, they need to win, and they will win, no matter what it takes. They do not doubt that they can achieve their goals. Instead, they know it's only a matter of doing the things they need to do to make their dreams come true. Many of you will never step on stage, but the same mindset applies. How badly do you want to put an inch on your arms, gain ten pounds, or get a six-pack? "Kind of" wanting it will not cut it. And how certain are you that your hard work will pay off? You had better be damn sure. If you lack confidence in your possibility of success, you will be holding back subconsciously and never putting out as much effort as you should be.

A final lesson you can take from the best pro's is that *they tend to work hardest on their weak points* in order to bring their physique closer to perfection. This is the opposite of what many bodybuilders and serious weight trainers do. They favor their best bodyparts, the ones that grow fastest and are the most fun to train. They tend to avoid or give short shrift to their training for areas that are more challenging. This only ensures that their physiques become more and more out of balance. How many guys have you seen with big arms and chests, and skinny legs? How many times does a guy look good from the front, but has no back development? How many legs look impressive from the front, but then the guy turns to the side and you see he has no hamstrings? If you are just trying to look good for the beach or the nightclub, that's fine and you can do what you like. But if you really want to have a balanced and proportionate physique like the pro's, you have to take it easy on your strong points and really prioritize your weak points.

To reach any degree of success in bodybuilding, it has to be nothing less than a lifestyle. I didn't say that it has to consume your entire life and define who you are as a person, but it does have to be as much a part of your life as waking up, breathing, and going to the bathroom. You don't only train when you are in the mood. You train when you are scheduled to train and you arrange your schedule around it. You don't eat the right foods only occasionally or when you are starving. Food is nothing more than fuel that you have to continually supply your body with at regular intervals to aid muscle recovery and repair.

So now it's established that the pro's don't really have any secrets. They train just like most other bodybuilders, they eat the same foods, and they even use the same exact supplements and drugs as many other thousands of men and women out there that identify themselves as bodybuilders. They look so much better than the average bodybuilder partly because of gifted genetics, and partly due to a tremendous drive and discipline that is also fairly rare.

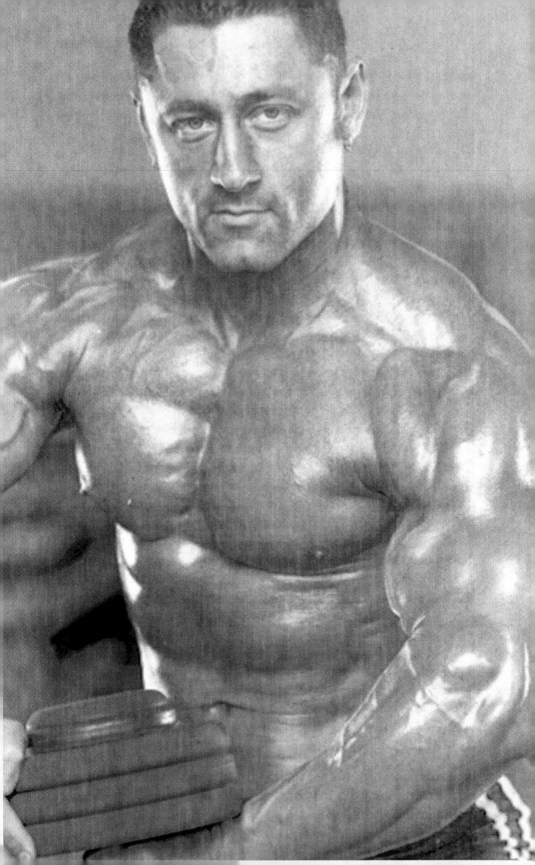

08

SUMMING UP

In this book, I have tried to give you an overview of much of what I've learned in the 25 years I have been building my own body, and in the nearly two decades I have worked in the industry of bodybuilding. In the end, you have to be your own teacher and your own student. Never strive to stop learning, as this is the true secret to being the best bodybuilder you can be. The day you decide you know it all is the day I guarantee you stop improving. Read everything you can. Talk, discuss, debate, experiment, these are the real secrets. Are you a real bodybuilder, or do you want to be one? The ball is in your court now and your journey is in progress. Travel it well. Never be afraid to ask for assistance or directions, and offer them when you can too. Just as everywhere else in life, you get back what you put into it. Don't get discouraged when progress isn't as fast as you would like. It never is. Just think of every hard workout and every good meal as another small step that gets you ever closer to your goals. One day you look back and can't believe how far you've come, as it seemed so many times you weren't getting anywhere. Above all else, remember these phrases:

"The more you know, the more you grow."

"Train hard, train smart, and never give up."

I wish you all the best of luck and God Bless.

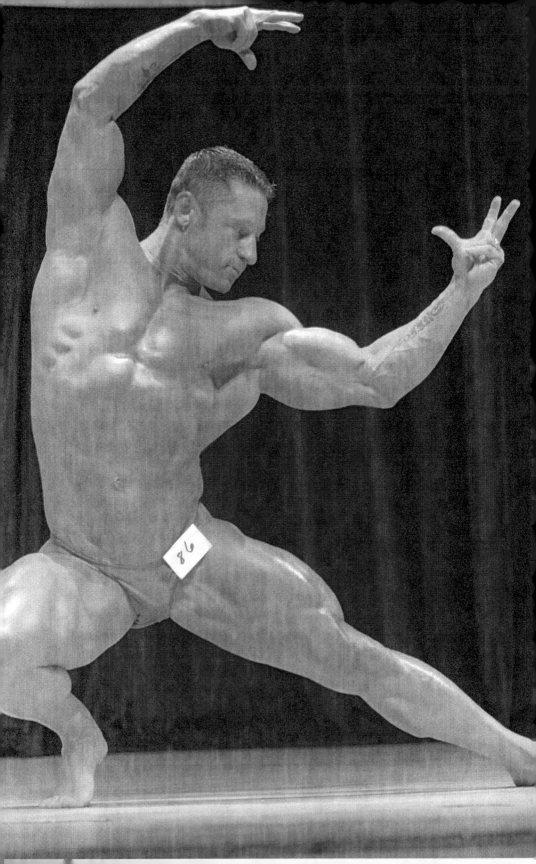

ACKNOWLEDGEMENTS

Thanks to my late parents, Alan and Ruth Harris, for raising me.

Thanks to my wife Janet, for putting up with me since that day we met in the fall of 1989. You keep me grounded on planet Earth and save me from myself.

Thanks to Lou Zwick of American Sports Network for getting me started in this crazy industry.

Thanks to John Balik and Steve Holman at *Ironman* magazine, for being the first to publish me and for keeping me on board ever since 1992. Thanks to the others that have allowed me to keep from having to work a 'real job,' Steve Blechman of *Muscular Development* and Bob Kennedy of *Musclemag International* and *REPS*. I don't even want to imagine what I would be doing right now if I weren't a writer.

Thanks to all the people that inspired me to be a bodybuilder, too numerous to name. Some were just kids at school with a little bit of muscle that I envied, others were pro wrestlers and Mr. Olympia winners. They all had an impact and made me want to change my body no matter what it took.

Thanks to the late Don "The Ripper" Ross, the craziest and most passionate man I ever knew, for inspiring me to take my own passions for the sport and for writing and to make a living at it.

And finally, thanks to all my readers and fans. You guys make it all worthwhile. If I have been able to motivate and teach, I know that those I have impacted will go on to do the same. We are all just part of one big never-ending chain.